HOMOEOPATHI
OF CHILDREN'

HOMOEOPATHIC TREATMENT OF CHILDREN'S AILMENTS

Remedies for Common Complaints

by

Dr E.A. Maury

Translated from the French by
Geoffrey A. Dudley B.A.

THORSONS PUBLISHERS LIMITED
Wellingborough, Northamptonshire

Published in France as
Soignez vos enfants par l'homoéopathie
© Jean-Pierre Delarge, Editions du Jour, Paris, 1975
First published in England 1978
Second Impression 1981
Third Impression 1982

© THORSONS PUBLISHERS LIMITED 1978

This book is sold subject to the condition that it shall not, by way of trade or otherwise, be lent, re-sold, hired out, or otherwise circulated without the publisher's prior consent in any form of binding or cover other than that in which it is published and without a similar condition including this condition being imposed on the subsequent purchaser.

ISBN 0 7225 0418 7

Printed and bound in Great Britain

CONTENTS

PREFACE

The therapeutic action of a remedy is based on the principle of similarity. This is the very foundation of homoeopathic medicine, the principles of which will be developed in the first part of this book, and is rightly applicable to the young child for various reasons.

Provided his biological environment has not been saturated during his intra-uterine life with poisonous drugs, alcohol, or tobacco originating from the mother, the child is like a soil, free from all polution, on which the Hahnemann remedy will exert a decidedly beneficial influence

Later on, during his early years, his small and still fragile organism will be subjected to attack from alien proteins with varying degrees of success. These are introduced through the medium of the numerous vaccines which are now available to parents. In the therapeutic part of this book I shall describe the homoeopathic medicines capable of acting as antidotes to the harmful and sometimes allergy-producing effects of even a mild form of these toxic microbes.

The young child can readily be compared to a young animal still free from any contamination by toxins.

Of course, there is no question of neglecting the often important role which can be played by hereditary factors transmitted by the genes; I shall return to it a little further on. To it can be attributed the appearance of disease symptoms which may take root as early as the first few months of life. Even in an organism not yet impaired by drugs or anything else, hereditary factors are the source of organic malformations or functional disorders which are sometimes irreversible. This question, however, cannot be answered in a book such as this, which is really intended for parents wishing to find a speedy preventive or curative remedy for a whole range of minor ailments or everyday complaints which can, to begin with at least be treated without consulting a doctor.

But, to revert to the comparison made above between the child and the young animal, my experience over more than forty years practice (although not as a vet) has led me to conclude that the Hahnemann remedy often works in a spectacular way on our animal friends, dogs or cats, indeed even on larger animals. I could cite many examples.

What must be remembered in this connection is that in both cases the practitioner is moving into virgin territory, on which the homoeopathic granule exerts an action considered to be independent of all suggestion. For how many times have we been assured that, for homoeopathy to act in the curative sense, it was first necessary to believe in its efficacy?

My forty-three years of day-to-day practice have, through the results obtained with young patients, enabled me to refute any apparent truth that there might be in this idea.

To come back once more to the question of the influence exerted by heredity on a yet unblemished organism, we can leave aside the cases of attack by toxins which have been considered above. However, in the young human being's biological balance-sheet, we shall have to take into account the existence of hereditary traits derived from immediate or remote ancestors, for example, in the shape of arthritic and rheumatoid tendencies or pathological saturations resulting from various microbial germs.

These pathogenic factors transmitted by the genes will give the child certain reactive tendencies which will affect two elements that the homoeopathic doctor must take into account in his clinical diagnosis and medicinal prescription, i.e., *constitution* and *temperament*.

In his clinical examination, the homoeopathic doctor will aim to determine his patient's typology, that is, his morphological characteristics which will be expressed by the two factors mentioned above. In fact, an individual's *constitution* is a function of the very shape of the skeleton and of the relations between its different parts, which remain fixed all through life: on the other hand, the *temperament* is a potential physiological state, but modified according to circumstances or shaped by individual peculiarities on the physical and mental planes.

To borrow an expression from Léon Vannier, who was our master in homoeopathy, it can be said that *constitution* is 'what is', *temperament* 'what is becoming'.

In an essentially practical work like this, one cannot develop at length everything that needs to be known about these two elements and their different clinical expressions. However, to give only a single example to explain why a homoeopathic medicine remains strictly individualized and varies in its prescription according to the patient's constitution and temperament, let me cite the treatment of a complaint which, at least to begin with, is relatively straightforward, i.e., flu.

If the reader will refer to the therapeutic part of this book, he will notice that, in the treatment of the early pathological symptoms of this illness, according to the possible clinical signs of the acute illness, two different remedies are indicated for combating *inter alia* the rise in body temperature. In one case *Aconite* is chosen and in the other *Belladonna*.

Why, when in orthodox medicine it is usual to prescribe only aspirin? Because, even with the same ailment, the clinical signs noted in the sick youngster (and this is equally true of adults) will differ according to his constitution and temperament. In one, the temperature will be up, the skin will stay dry and burning, and the bout of flu will give rise to signs of anxiety. These are all symptoms which will point to *Aconite*. In someone else with the same illness, the temperature could be lower but accompanied by a great deal of sweating and a state of torpor. All these, then, are the signs amenable to the prescription of *Belladonna*.

Of course, the mother cannot be expected to be deeply knowledgeable about the constitution and temperament of her offspring. The homoeopathic doctor consulted at the time will be able to enlighten her on this subject and guide her in his further prescriptions. But, by the example given above, I wish simply to make her understand why, for the same illness, she will have a choice among several remedies – according to the symptoms she has observed.

I have prepared this book exclusively for use with the child – from the very moment of conception, through his intra-uterine life, and up to the time of puberty.

For the various minor complaints and everyday illnesses without serious features, the mother will find the remedy or remedies all through the following pages. They will suit the circumstances and , I repeat, the particular character of the symptoms which are present. Moreover, in the first part of the book I shall recall the essential facts which should be known about homoeopathic medicine, its ease of application and its advantages.

Finally, to be as complete as possible in this brief study of ailments likely to afflict the child, it seemed to me useful to devote a special chapter to the functional disorders which the youngster can encounter during his years at school. For the school-child they often represent a difficult obstacle to surmount, to say nothing of the parents' very understandable concern over the set-backs experienced by their progeny. Here again, the suggested homoeopathic treatments can bring a happy solution to these problems while the patient is waiting for a medical or psychological opinion, as the case may be.

To conclude this foreword, I trust that any youngster treated in this way may quickly regain his health without his growth and development being harmed by abuse from the drugs with which today he tends to be force-fed.

I
HOMOEOPATHIC PRINCIPLES

INTRODUCTION

The ever more pronounced abuse of synthetic drugs belongs to our present way of life, which is based on the principle that inflation involves only economic factors. Like the frog in the fable who wanted to look like the ox, everything today is over-inflated. Without going outside the bounds of medicine, the only discipline about which I can speak with a certain authority, one has only to see the number of medications listed on a single allopathic prescription to prove this point. To be precise, it is fair to say that very often the patient himself judges his doctor only in relation to how large a sum of money he will have to lay out at the chemist's, even if it is just for an ordinary head cold.

It will be argued, with good reason, that the money spent by the patient may be generously repaid to him by the Social Security; so, for the person concerned, the financial problem does not exist from a practical point of view. Yet – and this is where the crunch comes – more than half the products prescribed are going to end up in the dutbin. This is clear proof that the patient really needed only the remaining half of the drugs to overcome his pathological symptoms.

The homoeopathic doctor, on the other hand, is more restrained with his prescriptions, and perhaps that is why his form of therapeutic assistance is still so little known and only rarely appreciated. His prescriptions are not expensive; *a priori*, therefore, the remedies which he advises must have for the outsider a value in keeping with the small amount of money which the patient lays out.

I have stressed the economic aspect of therapy, for, as stated above, in the mind of many patients a remedy which is expensive is a remedy which works. Well displayed, attractively packaged and brightly coloured, accompanied by persuasive directions for use, its favourable psychological impact will go halfway towards a cure.

By contrast, our humble granules are not much to look at compared with their big brothers of traditional medicine; yet they work, and in the following chapters I shall develop the reasons why you can put your trust in them. Besides, for pregnant women and also for the foetus and the child, taking them occasionally or regularly involves neither poisoning nor habituation, which are always to be feared with synthetic products.

1. WHAT IS HOMOEOPATHY?

A very large number of works have already been devoted to homoeopathic medicine during the century or more that it has been in existence and yet this therapeutic discipline still remains misunderstood, not in its practical applications but rather in the very terms of its definition.

People have tried to use an image to express the spirit of the Hahnemann method by relying purely and simply on the Greek etymology of the term; namely, to treat sickness with sickness. If you accept this fallacy, you may as well say that the treatment of a head cold caught in winter through exposure to cold consists in exposing yourself a second time to the rigours of the elements to achieve a cure. This interpretation, propagated especially by disparagers of our therapy, is nothing short of childish.

Let me then reinstate the truth.

Definition

Homoeopathy is a method of therapy (and I emphasize these terms) which consists of giving the patient, in very diluted and previously *dynamized* doses, the animal, vegetable, or mineral product which, in high or toxic doses, causes the same symptoms as those seen in the illness treated and which will therefore act as a remedy.

Examples

Better than long academic discussions, a few examples will lead to greater understanding of this technique of medicinal application, which is based on both objective signs and subjective sensations or impressions experienced by the patient.

Through having experienced them himself, everybody is aware of the purgative properties of calomel. We know that, given in a one gramme dose, this salt causes an attack of diarrhoea which lasts several hours. The final stools passed by the subject contain no more than mucus, the evacuation of which is painful, and the patient has the impression of never having finished emptying his bowels. Consequently, to obey the principle of similarity which will be taken up later, the homoeopathic doctor, confronted by a patient with diarrhoea, will prescribe that same remedy. This is especially true if the diarrhoea assumes the same characteristics as those determined by the massive absorption of calomel (as, for example, in cases of dysentery). But he will prescribe it for his patient in infinitesimal doses (and under its Latin name of *Mercurius dulcis*) in order to achieve healing of the intestinal inflammation.

Here is another example. In traditional doses, Ipecac is known to lead to the onset of vomiting. The subject who has ingested it experiences waves of sickness, feels poorly and throws up, although his tongue remains clean – a characteristic which represents one of the 'modalities' of the homoeopathic remedy *Ipecac*. So, when the homoeopathic doctor comes across a patient afflicted with nausea and vomiting, whose tongue remains clean regardless, he will prescribe *Ipecac* in infinitesimal doses, and this will have the effect of quickly arresting the symptoms reported.

And a final example: taken in too large a quantity, black coffee causes in most people restlessness, nervous irritation, hypersensitivity, intensification of mental activity and leads eventually to insomnia. Therefore, when faced with reactive phenomena of this kind (even if they are not due to the absorption of coffee), one will do well to take dilutions of coffee (*Coffea*) in order to put everything right again.

The three examples cited above throw light on the value of the 'tripod' on which the whole homoeopathic edifice rests, namely, *similarity, individualization* of the remedy, and, last, the *micro-dose*.

Here, as in the whole of the universe, which is perfect balance reflected in human balance, we rediscover the *trinity*, omnipresent in the midst of all expressions and all manifestations.

2. THE HOMOEOPATHIC TRIPOD

My aim in this chapter is to clarify what it is advisable to know about each of the three elements which constitute the very basis of Hahnemann therapeutics.

Similarity

As one of its bases, homoeopathy rests on the practical application of the law of similarity formulated by Hippocrates, some three hundred years before our era, in the following terms: 'Disease is produced by like things, and by the like things which one has the patient take, the latter returns from disease to health ...' And a little further on he adds: '... fever is suppressed by what produces it and produced by what suppresses it.'

Example of Quinine

The founder of homoeopathy, Samuel Hahnemann (1755-1833), started with these data and tested on himself the effects of Peruvian bark, taking it in measurable and regularly increasing doses over a certain period of time. He soon experienced all the symptoms of what it was agreed to call at that time marsh fever, now known as malaria; these took the form of a high temperature with shivers and an internal sensation of intense cold, the whole accompanied by chattering of the teeth, copious sweating, and pains in the joints.

Pathogenesis

Now, this same medicinal principle was already being used by the doctors of the time to fight symptoms of this type. It was seen as confirmation of the Hippocratic proposition which has been quoted above. But, by reducing more and more the dose of quinine used and then applying it to himself with a therapeutic aim, Hahnemann was able to demonstrate on himself first the lessening, then the disappearance, of the symptoms artificially produced by taking powerful doses of the product. This finding encouraged the young doctor, as he then was, to extend this same type of experiment to a certain number of other vegetable substances, then mineral ones, and finally animal substances.

Thus, thanks to this type of research carried out on man himself and not on animals, and given the name of *pathogenesis*, homoeopathy has been progressively enriched by a considerable number of pharmacodynamic observations, which have later been put to clinical use.

Similarity and Vaccination

Does not this principle of similarity find its confirmation in the very action of vaccination? We know that cowpox immunizes man against smallpox. The work of Louis Pasteur, who was a research chemist and biologist, has marked a turning-point in the history of medicine. For, perhaps without realizing it, this scientist applied the same law of similarity by introducing into modern therapeutics vaccines and serums, auto-serotherapy and auto-haemotherapy. To prevent rabies or to cure it with the help of the rabies virus is a striking example of the healing 'of disease by disease'. Could Pasteur have been a homoeopath without knowing it?

Individualization

The choice of homoeopathic remedy must, therefore, be specifically adapted to the sick person. That is, Hahnemann therapy does not include in its pharmacopoeia what is conveniently called the 'cure–all'.

Such is the second basis on which the method rests.

Modalities

The symptoms presented or experienced by the patient are his alone, regardless of the disease with which he is afflicted. As pointed out above, the sufferer reacts in some way to the onslaught of the disease according to his own temperament or constitution. This is why, after close questioning and a full clinical examination, he would be prescribed the remedy or remedies whose experimental characteristics correspond as nearly as possible to those expressed on the pathological level. This is what is called the *modalities* of the remedy.

Examples

To clarify my statement, let me take the example of subjects afflicted with, or in pain from, acute or chronic rheumatic attacks. One will tell you that he feels pain in his joints at the least movement but, on the other hand, when he is resting these pains disappear. Another will be stiff on waking or after a certain period of more or less prolonged immobility, whereas on walking or taking exercise he will be relieved.

These, then, are two different 'modalities' which imply the prescription of two different types of remedy, even for the same kind of illness.

'Signs'

The search for 'signs' is why the homoeopathic doctor questions and examines his patient so long and so searchingly. It is done with the aim of discovering the greatest number of pathological 'signs' peculiar to the patient himself; they will designate the corresponding 'like' remedy, according to the principle of similarity which has been explained in an earlier section.

I cannot leave this subject without recalling and summarizing here what L. Wurmser stated in the course of a paper read at the 26th Congress of Homoeopathic Medicine in May, 1967.

Variations of the 'Signs'

From the medical point of view, homoeopathy has, since Hahnemann, undergone many changes and important innovations, and it is towards a better understanding of the therapeutic action of the remedies, and to a better understanding of their individualization, that medical research must now be directed.

In fact, therapy by the 'identical', to use a more precise term, compels us more and more to adopt treatment by 'isopaths'. These are remedies still more plainly individualized since they are prepared from diseased strains taken from the ailing person himself (secretions, excretions, pathological products, etc.).

In conclusion, one can say with Wurmser that, through the importance which it gives to individual reactions, homoeopathy is a medicine for the whole man; through the richness and variety of its materia medica it permits effective intervention to re-establish a temporarily disturbed biological balance.

The effect of therapy is found to be even more remarkable in the young subject, whose organism has not yet been polluted by earlier medicinal poisons.

The Micro-dose

Homoeopathy has long been reproached for the infinitesimal quantities of its medicines, whatever the treatment. In the positive results obtained (for they do exist), people have tried to see solely the action of suggestion on the patient's part. I have already given my opinion on this subject. Besides, under the impetus of recent discoveries and thanks to the progress of biochemistry and microphysics, it is recognized that a minute dose of medicine can still be detected up to the Hahnemann ninth hundredth (9c). To understand properly the full importance of this figure and the significance that it can have, one should recall the way in which homoeopathic remedies are prepared in order to obtain higher and higher dilutions, i.e., medicines in the core of which the active principle is less and less condensed.

Preparation of the Remedy

If , for example, you start with a mother tincture of a product and wish to obtain a first centesimal dilution (1c), you mix a single drop of it in ninety-nine drops of alcohol. To obtain the second centesimal (2c), you take a single drop of the previous preparation, mixing it again with ninety-nine drops of alcohol, and so on until the ninth centesimal (9c), which has been discussed above, is obtained. Succussion at all stages is very important.

Small globules with a pure lactose base are immersed in the solution containing the remedy and by this 'impregnation', which was greatly valued by Hahnemann, they are then transformed into active medicinal granules. For the low and average dilutions, granules which weigh twenty to the gramme are used and, for doses of 7c, 9c and over, globules which weigh three hundred and fifty to the gramme.

Impregnation of the granules is achieved by putting them in the solution for a few minutes, and then shaking the bottle to obtain consistency in the impregnation. They are subsequently dried out of the reach of dust.

Controlling the Dose

Control of the impregnation of the globules and granules has been achieved by pouring one drop of a coloured solution on one gramme of neutral samples, which established that there were some variations in the look and intensity of the coloration depending on the process of manufacture. Hence, so that a granule becomes truly medicinal and therefore therapeutically active after impregnation, its manufacture must observe certain norms or presentation, solubility, absorption, preservation and size.

An experiment performed by Wurmser, already cited above, proves that a very weak dose of a chemical product can permit the administration of a toxic product. If guinea-pigs are poisoned by giving them powerful enough doses of arsenic, only 37 per cent of the product is eliminated spontaneously; but, to reach a 42 per cent level of elimination, the experimenter gave these laboratory animals, previously poisoned with arsenic, infinitesimal doses of the same poison, i.e., arsenic in homoeopathic doses.

Two points are now established: first, the micro-dose, the third leg of the tripod, is effectively the basis of the Hahnemann medication, and, in the second place, it works in the same direction as the disease which has been artificially caused by absorption of the same product given in measurable doses.

Moreover, at the present time the infinitesimal dose is used in orthodox medicine in anti-allergic treatments, in which, to desensitize him, the patient is injected with active doses containing only a fifty-millionth part of the initial product.

3. CHARACTERISTICS OF HOMOEOPATHIC TREATMENT

Rapidity of Action

It is still currently put about that homoeopathy is a therapy whose action and efficacy make themselves felt only in the long run, solely in clinical cases which have been wrongly labelled, or in the course of chronic complaints. Contrary to this opinion, I can assert what my own experience has shown me countless times. This is that, provided that it is correctly prescribed according to the symptoms observed in the subject under treatment, the Hahnemann remedy evinces a speed of action and an efficacy at least equal, if not in many cases superior, to those which can be expected from medications currently in vogue.

One can even lay down as a law, of which I have many times ascertained the truth, that disease in its acute, virulent and episodic form (flu, for instance) progresses more rapidly towards cure and hence the duration of its morbid cycle grows that much shorter.

This feature is still more marked in the child, who, more so than the adult, responds rapidly to medication.

Universality

To reply once more to the major objection, namely that homoeopathy is a therapy which is effective because of the process of auto-suggestion, it will be recalled that this medicine is supremely adaptable. It works just as well in very young children and in animals, both of whom are completely insensitive to the influence of preconceived ideas. In the same way, the spontaneous opening of a boil or abscess, to give just one example, under the combined effect of remedies like *Hepar Sulphur* or *Myristica* belongs to the realm of real facts, easily verifiable by anyone of good faith.

So it can be said that the objection about suggestibility does not stand up to the facts any more than does that of the inefficacy of the remedies.

Harmlessness

It hardly seems useful to dwell on the total absence of toxicity of homoeopathic remedies, since until recent years, the orthodox school had not acknowledged them to have any therapeutic value and had raised the objection that there were no active ingredients whatsoever in the preparations.

In this connection I shall not go over what has already been said in the previous chapter, in the section devoted to the study of the micro-dose, namely, that the active principle of the medication is experimentally demonstrable even in the highest dilutions.

It is not any the less true that the medicinal product used to obtain the remedy is found in such infinitesimal quantities that even its prolonged use runs no risk of causing any symptom of poisoning or allergy.

The subject concerned, especially if he is being treated for the first time by homoeopathy, can be expected to exhibit incidental 'reactions' to the remedies prescribed. A cleansing crisis or toxic discharge may actually occur in the diseased organism, triggered off as a result of the medicinal action (which proves once again the reality of the therapeutic effect), but these 'crises' are in other respects absolutely harmless. We might even say they are beneficial since their occurrence is evidence that the organism is putting up a good defence. There is nothing unnatural about them and they are a powerful aid to the organism in its return to health.

In a sense we can put them in the same class with what are commonly called the 'thermal crises' which come on during a mineral-spa treatment.

Non-Addictiveness

Contrary to the effects of drugs used in orthodox practice, homoeopathic medicines do not produce the phenomenon known as 'habituation'. This is due to the organism's condition of pharmaceutical saturation, which occurs regardless of the use and duration of the prescription.

A Hahnemann remedy, accurately prescribed according to

the principles of the method and particularly when prescribed at the right time – and I shall stress below the value of the 'moment' for taking it – always works, producing every time, under the same pathological conditions, the same curative effects.

Hence there is no call to fear, as there is with chemotherapeutic or antibiotic drugs, a saturation of the organism and a therapeutic shock depending more on the drug poisoning than on a favourable organic reaction to the progress of the disease.

Therapeutic Value

Besides establishing that, through the effect of correctly prescribed homoeopathic remedies, the patient rapidly regains his health, there is an enormous amount of skill in the art of prescription itself, which demands an exact knowledge of the 'moment' when it is right to give such and such a remedy.

One notices that, under the influence of the medication and especially in cases of acute children's illnesses, the pathological development is quite rapid. The symptoms present in the young patient in the evening, for example, can be seen to be different from those in evidence the following morning. As a result, the prescription will need to be changed, since the pathological signs, the importance of which has been seen above and which would decide the choice of a first remedy at the start of the day, will have disappeared. Under the curative influence of this first medication, they will have made way for other developmental symptoms of the complaint, and these are going to necessitate prescribing other remedies in harmony – or, better, 'in similarity' – with the signs noted or experienced by the patient. The illness running its course will be seen to 'live', as it were; only pertinent observation of the symptoms presented by the patient will allow the homoeopath to revise his prescription to make a change beneficial for the patient and which will help him to take a fresh step towards recovery.

4. APPLICATION OF THE TREATMENT

The standard homoeopathic remedy, which can be obtained from homoeopathic pharmacies (*see Appendix*), comes in the form of small granules or pilules (according to size) of pure lactose, impregnated with the active substance which gives its name (in Latin) to the medicine. In an earlier section I have stressed the technique used in the preparation of the remedies by specialized laboratories. Further, in addition to the name of the product, each remedy carries on the label the level of dilution (3c and upwards), which corresponds to the number of successive transfers of the active principle into the diluting agent, the latter generally being pure alcohol.

Choice of Dilutions

Some homoeopathic laboratories supply the same remedies to the same standards of dilution, but in liquid form. In this case, their prescription and dosage belong to the doctor, who is the sole judge of how many drops to use and their daily frequency.

In most cases of childhood complaints of an acute character, the study of which will constitute the most important part of this book, it is preferable to turn to remedies in a low dilution, usually the Hahnemann fourth centesimal, labelled 6c on the tube of pilules. In fact, clinical experience has proved that, the more the disease presents a severe or acute character (high temperature, stubborn symptoms, etc), the more desirable it is to select a remedy in a low dilution, i.e., one whose active principle is still relatively close to the mother tincture from which the chemist started in preparing it.

Choice of Remedies

If the symptoms change in character, the prescription then needs to be modified. That is why we ask the mother to keep a close eye on the development of the illness in her small patient. Hence, starting with a new remedy selected in accordance with the new signs determined and indicated by the 'moment' of the illness, the physician will prepare a new solution in the same conditions and doses; the frequency of application also remains the same. Of course, immediately on improvement of the pathological condition, the regular doses of the solution will be spaced out by omitting one or two hours, depending on circumstances.

All these recommendations will be repeated in connection with the treatment of each of the complaints looked at in the clinical part of this work. If, on the other hand, the homoeopath is concerned with young patients whose state of health does not call for rest in bed, he can then give the indicated granules orally. The patient can let three or four units of the selected or prescribed medicine melt on the tongue every two to three hours during the day, not exceeding, however, the total amount of ten to twelve granules of the same remedy per day.

Dosage

The preceding section has raised the question of the medicinal solution prepared from the remedy or remedies indicated to be given in case of need. I will repeat this point once again to make it quite clear.

As the most convenient way of administering the therapy to the young patient, I advise letting the selected granules dissolve in a glass of pure water (Vittel or Evian, for instance) at the rate of ten granules for a single remedy. Once these granules have dissolved (this takes about twenty to twenty-five minutes), a tablespoonful of the solution should be given every hour to a child over seven years old. For infants one would recommend instead a teaspoonful of the medicinal solution and only every other hour.

Auxiliary Medications

Administering or taking homoeopathic remedies naturally does not exclude all the external medications which are necessary in individual cases.

Moreover, in the therapeutic part of this book and in connection with symptoms affecting the skin or mucous membranes, mention will be made of the application of salves or ointments containing active principles of vegetable origin taken from the Hahnemann pharmacopoeia.

All these prescriptions may perhaps appear a bit old-fashioned, but they are no less effective for that. This is true whether they come in the form of poultices, cupping-glasses, mustard plasters, wet packs, gargles, etc., or used as vegetable laxatives and sudorific (perspiration) or diuretic (urine) infusions, providing the taking of which is always indicated in the course of fevers.

Clinical Index

For the greatest convenience in the practical use of this book, I have reviewed as succinctly as possible the commonest complaints likely to occur in a child's life; but they are ones which are not serious enough to require sending for the doctor immediately.

II
THE CHILD IN THE WOMB

INTRODUCTION

If I were to claim to develop at this point certain ideas about genetics, they might, although going right to the heart of the problem, imply metaphysical aspects which it is not my purpose to introduce in an essentially practical work; yet one can consider that the future human being possesses a biological entity right from the moment of conception.

Therefore, a reminder about prenatal eugenics does not seem out of place.

What can be understood by this term?

On consulting the definition given in the *Larousse* dictionary, we find that eugenics is the science dealing with the whole range of conditions favourable to the reproduction of the human species.

Consequently, the study and knowledge of this factor will enable us to bring to the child (from the mother's breast) the full complement of materials necessary for his growth as well as the means to be used in detoxifying him from his pathological heredity.

According to the most recent statistics, there is a constant increase in the number of children who are abnormal, mentally handicapped, or otherwise maladjusted. A preventive therapy recommended to the mother by the homoeopathic paediatrician is, therefore, imposed from the first month of pregnancy. In fact, in the nucleus of its primitive cells the embryo potentially contains the stigmas transmitted by the forebears. These will manifest themselves in the foetus during its intra-uterine life, to appear next in the first few months of the baby's normal life, once he has left the mother's womb.

So one can predicate that, for the whole duration of

pregnancy, the future adult in miniature ought to be the object of preventive care through the mother who bears him.

My aim, however, in the pages which follow is not to look at the judicious handling of pregnancy from the moment of conception to the end of confinement. A very large number of works have been published on this subject and to these the mother-to-be will naturally refer.

I wish to mention here only the appropriate medicinal principles taken from the homoeopathic pharmacopoeia and capable of being applied to the foetus. It is, therefore, simply a matter of giving practical advice and of indicating some popular remedies intended for the mother-to-be, for her own mistakes about hygiene or the occurrence of some of her discomforts might upset the child's biological balance during the nine months of his life in the womb.

Then again, one will at the same time insist on the main medicines which are intended for the foetus itself and which will help to turn it into a strong and healthy baby.

As in most of my works dealing with practical homoeopathy, I have, for the reader's convenience, again adopted here the alphabetical listing which enables the name of the complaint or the failure of hygiene to be easily found at the same time as the remedy or remedies to be used in either case.

But, as stated above, there can be no question of giving long descriptions of diseases and exhaustive therapeutic considerations: these can fall only within the competence of the physician or paediatrician.

My aim is thus to remain on firm, everyday ground. Yet I cannot pass over in silence the role which genetics will play in modifications of normal or pathological traits transmitted by the parents.

Of course, it is not always easy to foresee the influence which hereditary factors may have, threatening to handicap the child during his life. At one time the family doctor, a true practitioner of the art of healing, could, from his knowledge of the parents' medical histories, recognize in most cases the disorders likely to befall the child; but today, even though medicine has made immense progress, it has become almost impossible for the practitioner and even more so for the specialist, although he is a veritable fount of knowledge, to see into the biological future of the new-born.

On the other hand, the homoeopathic doctor is a traditionalist bound by his Hippocratic oath. With his knowledge of temperaments and constitutions, of which mention has been made in the first part of the book, he is qualified to predict the pathological future of the adult in embryo and avert any adverse consequences as far as is possible. More will be said about this in the second part of this book, which applies exclusively to the child in the womb and the mother who carries him.

CLINICAL INDEX

A number of complaints or mistakes of hygiene threaten to influence the biological balance of the pregnant woman throughout her pregnancy. Among them we have selected those which could have repercussions on the well-being of the foetus, and we have suggested certain remedies to mitigate their drawbacks.

Of course, in the event of worsening or clinical complications, the mother-to-be cannot be too strongly advised to call upon her doctor's help.

ALBUMINURIA

During pregnancy it can happen that a woman may find her condition complicated by the presence of albumin in her urine.

This protein factor is evidence of some insufficiency of renal (kidney) function. It occurs under the influence of causes which it is the doctor's task to clarify and which, if not treated, threaten to bring on attacks of eclampsia (coma and convulsions). These are naturally prejudicial to the well-being of the foetus.

As soon as albumin appears in the urine, independently of salt reduction, always act according to the homoeopathic principle of similarity. Depending on the symptoms noted in the pregnant woman, one will have a choice between two remedies.

Apis mellifica 6c (phial)

Symptoms: Albuminuria is accompanied by the existence of a partial or general oedema (excess of fluid) affecting the mucous or serous membranes and complicated by burning or stabbing pains; worth noting are the absence of thirst and the desire for cold milk.

Doses: 3 granules four times a day between meals.

Helonia dioica 6c (phial)

Symptoms: Apart from the presence of albumin in the urine, due in most cases to a dropped stomach affecting the kidneys, the pregnant woman complains of heaviness in the pelvic region with fatigue and exhaustion; it can be said that she 'feels her womb,' and this sensation is communicated to the sacral region.

Dosage: 3 granules four times a day between meals.

ALCOHOL (Excess of)

Naturally, the mother-to-be cannot be too strongly recommended to refrain strictly from taking any alcohol (aperitif or liqueur) during her pregnancy. But a good-quality red wine, in particular Médoc, can supply mineral and vitamin-enriched elements which will be as favourable to the mother as to the foetus.

However, in the event of occasional or habitual alcoholism, there is a remedy which can act as an antidote to the toxic effects; what is more, its regular use will contribute to combating the desire for alcoholic drinks.

Quercus glandium spiritus 3x (bottle)

Symptoms: A thick head with sudden flushes and a tendency to attacks of dizziness.

Dosage: 20 drops in a little water before main meals.

ANTIBIOTICS (Antidote to)

The current pharmacopoeia uses and especially abuses antibiotics. These are certainly indicated in many cases, but their prescription must recognize limits; failing this, their beneficial effects become in the long run harmful to the mother's organism and all the more to the foetus's. The latter, once it has developed and left the mother's womb, runs the risk of becoming allergic to this type of medication if applied in the event of microbial infection, even an ordinary and benign one. But it can also become, as it were, 'mithridatized'.[1] This implies either a fresh choice of antibiotics or an increase in the normal dose, with the disadvantages which this solution entails.

Hence the mother-to-be who has had to use antibiotics during her pregnancy will be well advised to take a homoeopathic antidote.

Hepar sulphur 6c (phial)

Symptoms: Homoeopathic experience has shown that, applied either during or after antibiotic treatment, this remedy strengthens the female patient's resistance to the secondary effects of antibiotic medication.

To the element *Sulphur* contained in this medicine can be attributed its often powerful action of organic detoxification and drainage of waste products.

Dosage: 5 granules twice a day between meals.

DECREASE OF CALCIUM IN TEETH AND BONES

From the early days of pregnancy the future mother brings to the future baby the nutritive and anabolic elements indispensable to his growth. Among these elements calcium salts make a contribution which plays an all-important role in building the bony skeleton.

Independently of foods rich in mineral substances, a supplementary contribution of calcium compounds can only be an asset to both mother and child during the intra-uterine period.

Two homoeopathic remedies are then to be recommended.

Avena sativa 1x (bottle)

Symptoms: Nervous fatigue with bouts of insomnia and lack of general tone.

Dosage: 20 drops in a little water before meals.

Calcareous compounds 6c (powder)

Symptoms: Marked decrease of calcium in teeth and bones

[1] A reference to Mithridates, king of Pontus (*c.* 120-63 B.C.), who is said to have made himself immune to poisons by taking gradually increasing doses of them. — *Trans.*

with sensation of cold penetrating right to the bones, particularly at the level of the leg and the foot.

Dosage: 2 or 3 measures dry under the tongue before the two main meals.

HAEMORRHAGES

In a pregnant woman any loss of blood, regardless of its cause, may have adverse consequences for the growth of the foetus and later for the health of the future baby due to an impoverishment of red corpuscles. Two homoeopathic remedies will then be indicated, depending on the clinical aspects which these haemorrhages may assume.

Arnica 3x (bottle)

Symptoms: This remedy is indicated in all cases where the loss of blood is directly related to an injury; the whole body is painful, as though it had been beaten; even at night the bed appears hard and the patient cannot find a good place to lie on.

Dosage: 15-20 drops in a little water three or four times a day.

China 6c (phial)

Symptoms: Repeated and prolonged haemorrhages which affect the mucous membranes or the orifices of the body produce in a pregnant woman a severely anaemic condition with a chilly sensation which reaches all through the body. The result is that the subject feels the least draught.

Dosage: Dissolve 15 granules in a glass of water and give a dessertspoonful every half-hour.

HEREDITARY INFLUENCES

It is rather hard for the mother-to-be to predict the future of the foetus which she carries in her womb. Too many previous generations are already represented in the transmitted genes, and one is entitled to show ignorance of the merit and drawbacks of such influence. Yet, with the object of eliminating as far as possible the ever-present risks of heredity, which are, moreover, often ill defined, one will offer a suggestion to the pregnant woman. This is that, throughout her pregnancy, she should take the two remedies indicated below every fortnight.

Hydrastis 3x (bottle)

Symptoms: Called in homoeopathy a 'drainage' medicine, it affects particularly the mucous membranes, which react with a thick and yellowish discharge; this 'catarrhal' state is accompanied by extreme weakness and marked loss of weight.

Dosage: 15-20 drops before the two main meals.

'Sulphur iodatum 6c (phial)

Symptoms: Self-poisoning in women with tubercular heredity; chronic enlarged tonsils and skin irritation; tendency to herpes of the lips.

Dosage: 3 granules 3 times a day.

Still on the subject of hereditary influences and as already said in the previous pages, only the homoeopathic physician who has known the mother-to-be's family and antecedents for a long time can act with full knowledge of the case. His action will be all the more effective if he prescribes certain homoeopathic remedies known as 'biotherapeutic'; these are adapted to suspected or recognized hereditary factors.

MISCARRIAGE (Tendencies to)

In a certain number of cases of habitual tiredness or in the aftermath of a prolonged illness occurring in the pregnant woman, the pregnancy may be interrupted and the stillborn foetus expelled prematurely.

As a preventive measure, a homoeopathic medicine is capable of helping the mother-to-be and of enabling her to carry her pregnancy through normally.

Aletris farinosa 3x (bottle)

Symptoms: Intense fatigue with a sensation of heaviness in the lower part of the abdomen and false labour pains.

Dosage: 15-20 drops in a little water three or four times a day.

MISCARRIAGE (Threat of)

Without entering into details of complex pathology, we wish to remain on essentially practical ground. So before the arrival of the doctor sent for in this eventuality, we shall recommend a remedy which acts particularly in the uterus.

Sabina 6c (phial)

Symptoms: Bleeding from the womb may occur at the least movement; the blood is bright red and mixed with clots; the abdominal pains are violent and extend from the pubis to the sacrum.

Dosage: Dissolve 15-20 granules in a glass of water and give a dessertspoonful every 15-20 minutes.

MOVEMENTS OF THE FOETUS

This eventuality will concern the pregnant woman rather than the little being that she carries in her womb. Yet the foetal motor reactions can be thought of as threatening to upset both the mother and the baby to come.

With the object of improving this physiological condition and mitigating the drawbacks, one remedy is to be recommended.

Arnica 6c (phial)

Symptoms: The baby's movements can be particularly felt and are painful during the night; the pregnant woman has the totally subjective impression that 'the foetus is lying the wrong way.'

Dosage: 3 granules three or four times a day.

NAUSEA

This symptom, which is in some cases peculiar to the pregnant woman, does not directly involve the foetus; but in any case it is preferable to mitigate this drawback in the mother-to-be.

Cocculus 6c (phial)

Symptoms: Nausea accompanied by dizziness and hiccups; an empty feeling in the stomach with aversion to the ordinary smell of food.

Dosage: 3 granules every 15-20 minutes until feeling better.

TOBACCO (Antidote to)

The mother-to-be cannot be too strongly recommended to avoid the use of cigarettes. The poisons which they contain, whether nicotine or the residues of combustion, pass via the placenta into the foetal organism and thereby contribute to its toxic condition.

In this case two homoeopathic remedies are advised.

Caladium 6c (phial)

Symptoms: For the inveterate smoker who does not have the will-power to stop using the weed, this medicine serves as an antidote to the effects of tobacco. Sometimes it is even successful in modifying the need to have recourse to cigarettes.

Dosage: 3 granules three times a day.

Ignatia 6c (phial)

Symptoms: In the present case, the indication for this remedy will rest rather on the physio-pathological consequences of tobacco poisoning, in particular the aversion to tobacco smoke after too many cigarettes. From the sensory viewpoint, there is also an accompanying migraine, the painful character of which is peculiar to this remedy: the pregnant woman feels as if a nail were being driven into the side of her head.

Dosage: 3 granules three times a day.

VOMITING IN PREGNANCY

What has been said above about nausea in the pregnant woman can be repeated under this heading. These unpleasant symptoms do not directly affect the foetus, but nevertheless they threaten to alter its biological balance.

So it is desirable to mitigate this drawback and homoeopathically a remedy is indicated for just such an eventuality.

Ipecac 6c (phial)

Symptoms: The vomit, preceded by nausea, is mucous and resembles white of egg. It brings no relief; in fact, despite these gastric signs, the tongue stays clean and salivation is intense.

Dosage: 3 or 4 granules every half hour until the reactions stop.

III

THE SICK CHILD

INTRODUCTION

In the lines which follow we shall only recall what has already been said in the introduction to the second part of this work. But this time we shall have as our aim the occasional or emergency treatment of the minor complaints which may occur in the child from the day of his birth up to about the time of puberty.

Outside this period, which represents an important stage in the life of the future adult, we refer the mother to works dealing with the homoeopathic therapy of common illnesses of benign aspect which, at least at their onset, do not always call for medical attention.

But, before we recommend the therapy to be used in individual cases, it is as well to clarify what the affliction we meant to treat may represent.

Meaning of the illness

Reference has already been made above to the influence which heredity can have on the child's biological growth as early as the period of his intra-uterine existence.

Once he has been launched into the world, until the critical age of puberty, the little creature is going to present a whole series of more or less serious afflictions, classed under the general term of 'childhood diseases'. Most of these pathological occurrences must be considered as so many means of defence of the immature organism against the effects of the various hereditary stigmas transmitted by the parents.

One must never forget, as one is apt to do, that the disease, in whatever form it appears, is nothing but the culmination of acquired or inherited morbid conditions, against which the subject must protect himself with a view to preserving his biologcial wholeness.

Acute illness, such as appears in the child, will, therefore, be considered as a crisis of elimination and organic cleansing. Thus it represents a necessary stage to be gone through to purify the infant organism and so consolidate the health of the future adult.

Unfortunately, in our so-called 'scientific' and 'functional' age and in the name of a preventive measure based on ill-timed vaccinations applied systematically and blindly, the time for the cleansing crisis is put off, even if it isn't withheld.

Indeed, in the absence of these signs of disease, the mother congratulates herself on the apparent good health of her offspring. She has no idea, for no one has told her, that things will come inescapably to a head and the later they appear, the higher the cost.

The mother must be able to understand the meaning of these signs in the youngster, for, correctly treated by Hahnemann remedies, they will evince only a minimum of severity and complications.

Homoeopathic 'biotherapeutics'

Our attention could be called to the fact that preventive vaccinations have avoided the appearance of serious diseases which in the past have contributed to promoting infantile mortality.

It would be childish to deny it, more especially as the principle which is at the very root of these applications rests on the law of similarity, the basis of homoeopathy.

It is important, however, to avoid their excesses and to know their contra-indications; we have already given the reason for this in the previous section.

Nevertheless, the Hahnemann therapeutic arsenal puts a whole series of remedies at the doctor's disposal. Prepared like traditional vaccines from bacterial stocks, but more diluted and dynamized, they are known by the name of 'biotherapeutics'. Quite like traditional vaccines, they will find a use as prophylactics in the event of an epidemic or a threat of contagion. Their prescription and dosage, however, are at the practioner's discretion.

How to use the handbook

For the utmost convenience in handling this book, we have

reviewed, system by system, the minor, classic-type complaints which can affect or impair the immature organism's normal functioning.

To quote but one example, that of common disorders affecting the respiratory organs, we have given *inter alia* the homoeopathic treatment of sore throats, bronchitis, whooping-cough, flu, otitis (inflammation of the ear), coughs, and adenoids. It will be the same for complaints of the alimentary canal, the nervous system, and the skin. A special section is devoted to fever and fevers with rashes and another to certain disorders affecting the general condition which cannot be included in the above-mentioned classification.

Finally, we ask the mother to take careful note of the pathological signs which she finds in the child and to select the remedy or remedies according to the symptoms presented.

With the aim of confirming herself in her choice, she will refer to the last part of this manual. Under the title of 'Materia Medica,' this develops the pathogenesis of each of the remedies indicated for each of the diseases mentioned. As for the degree of dilution selected and the dose recommended, they are both shown for each of the medicines chosen.

1. RESPIRATORY ORGANS

ACUTE BRONCHITIS

An ordinary chill occurring in a frail youngster carries the risk of complications from inflammation of the bronchia.

Depending on the symptoms observed or presented, there will be a choice of three remedies.

Antimonium tartaricum 6c (phial)

Symptoms: The cough is accompanied by considerable wheezing due to accumulations of phlegm in the bronchia, but there is almost no expectoration. Breathing is noisy and difficult, the nostrils are dilated, and the sides of the nose move in and out in time with the movements of breathing.

Dosage: Dissolve 10 granules in a glass of water and give a dessertspoonful of the solution every hour.

Bryonia 6c (phial)

Symptoms: In this case, the cough is dry and spasmodic; it is aggravated by the slightest movement made by the young patient. He also complains of acute pains in the chest and has to hold his thorax firmly with both hands every time he coughs.

Dosage: Dissolve 10 granules in a glass of water and give a dessertspoonful of the solution every hour.

Ferrum phosphoricum 6c (phial)

Symptoms: This remedy is suitable at the very onset of bronchial inflammation; the cough is dry, spasmodic, painful, but it may be accompanied by expectoration which is sometimes streaked with blood; fever is always present and the pulse is rapid and weak.

Dosage: Dissolve 10 granules in a glass of water and give a dessertspoonful of the solution every hour.

ACUTE OTITIS

Inflammation of the middle ear is a condition frequently met with during childhood, whether it occurs spontaneously or whether it comes as a complication of an infection already attacking the upper respiratory tract.

A medical examination of the auditory ducts is the rule in this case, but meanwhile in the emergency case one's choice can be directed towards two remedies.

Aconitum 6c (phial)

Symptoms: Pain in the afflicted ear comes on abruptly after a chill, especially in dry weather. It is acute, unbearable, and more pronounced at night. The head is heavy; the child is restless and anxious; his skin is burning and dry and fever, which is often high, is accompanied by shivering.

Dosage: Dissolve 10 granules in a glass of water and give one tablespoonful of the solution every half-hour.

Ferrum phosphoricum 6c (phial)

Symptoms: This remedy is indicated right from the initial stage of otitis. The affected ear is the seat of attacks of violent pain characterized by throbbing – symptoms which are relieved by local applications of cold water.

The child is anxious, restless, and hypersensitive to noises.

The fever is accompanied by bouts of sweating which do not relieve the young patient.

Dosage: Dissolve 10 granules in a glass of water and give a tablespoonful of the solution every half hour.

ADENOIDS

The increase in volume of the glandular tissue which lines the back of the nose and the pharynx often represents a serious hindrance to the child's breathing and later on to his full physical and mental development.

It is indispensable to undertake a radical treatment, which must be handled by the paediatrician. But, in simple cases presenting no major complications, one can always advise here two remedies which will alleviate the drawbacks of this type of complaint.

Pulsatilla 6c (phial)

Symptoms: With this remedy, all the mucous membranes are affected. At the level of the upper respiratory tract, the secretions are thick, yellowish, and non-irritant. The right nostril is generally blocked and the sense of smell diminished. In the psychological sphere, the child is timid and emotional and cries for nothing.

Dosage: 3 granules four times a day between meals.

Silicea 6c (phial)

Symptoms: This remedy is indicated for children who have undergone too many inoculations or who have not taken them well. The organism then reacts by increasing the volume of glandular tissues, which are for protection against infection or viruses. The nose is stuffed up, the tonsils swollen, and swallowing remains difficult if not painful.

Dosage: 3 granules four times a day between meals.

ASTHMA

In this work, which is intended for family use, the complete treatment will not, of course, be given for this complaint, which is met with rather early in the child's life. Too many factors, as much biological as psychological, are taken into account in the origin of the disorder.

But a homoeopathic remedy to be applied right at the start of the attack will bring rapid relief to the little patient.

Sambucus nigra 3x (bottle)

Symptoms: The child wakes up abruptly in the middle of the night gasping for breath and has difficulty in breathing out; face and extremities are blue and the child is unable to lie with his head on the pillow.

Dosage: 20 drops in half a glass of water; give a teaspoonful of the solution every 10-15 minutes.

COLDS

The common head cold, which up to now has triumphantly resisted all forms of therapy, can be correctly treated and quickly arrested, thanks to homoeopathic treatment.

Always in accordance with the symptomatology established in the young patient, the mother will have a choice of two medicines.

Allium cepa 6c (phial)

Symptoms: Frequent sneezing accompaned by heavy nasal secretions which are watery and irritating to the nostrils and upper lip; this type of cold comes on particularly after exposure to cold and damp air.

Dosage: Dissolve 10 granules in a glass of water and give a dessertspoonful of the solution every hour.

Arsenicum album 6c (phial)

Symptoms: In this case the nasal secretions are watery and produce cold sores; they are accompanied by a sharp burning sensation at the level of the mucous membranes of the nose, which is blocked; sneezing does not bring any relief.

Dosage: Dissolve 10 granules in a glass of water and give a dessertspoonful of the solution every hour.

COUGHS

Many remedies can be selected from the homoeopathic arsenal to relieve the patient, more especially as this reflex symptom, which is due to irritation or inflammation of the mucous membranes of the respiratory system, has many causes and various clinical signs.

With a view to simplifying the mother's choice and prior to a medical opinion, if one is needed, three remedies will be given below, each corresponding to a different aspect of the cough.

Bryonia 6c (phial)

Symptoms: Usually originating in irritation of the trachea, the cough is dry, spasmodic and worse during the night. This forces the child to sit up in bed and grip the thorax; in fact, the least movement contributes further to worsening this reaction, as also does the fact of moving into too warm a room.

Dosage: Dissolve 10 granules in a glass of water and give a dessertspoonful of the solution every hour.

Antimonium tartaricum 6c (phial)

Symptoms: The choice of this remedy is dictated by the very nature of the cough; it is loose, for the bronchia are congested with phlegm, which the little patient brings up with difficulty and in too small amounts. Worth noting, too, is the fact that the cough improves if he lies on his right side.

Dosage: Dissolve 10 granules in a glass of water and give a dessertspoonful of the solution every hour.

Kali bichromicum 6c (phial)

Symptoms: The cough is set off by irritation at the point where the larynx starts; it is harrowing and metallic. The voice is hoarse and the sputum is yellowish, slimy, and copious. Sometimes the child complains of a pain beginning behind the breastbone, passing through the thorax, and going up to the shoulders.

Dosage: Dissolve 10 granules in a glass of water and give a dessertspoonful every hour.

FLU

There is often a tendency to confuse this illness with the common head cold, the treatment of which has been given in a previous section.

The flu virus, which is particularly active in cold and damp months, first attacks the nervous system. It is only secondarily that there appears symptoms affecting the respiratory organs, which are a preferred site for this pathogenic (disease forming) agent. That is why the first-aid treatment of this illness has been grouped in this chapter.

It is, therefore, a good idea for the mother to be able to recognize flu from the symptoms presented.

If the diagnosis is positive, she will have a choice of two remedies.

Eupatorium perfoliatum 6c (phial)

Symptoms: The young patient complains of aching and

stiffness involving bones and muscles; the eyeballs, too, are painful. The temperature is up, especially after waking in the morning; this is preceded by a sensation of intense thirst and accompanied by shivering.

Dosage: Dissolve 10 granules in a glass of water and give a dessertspoonful of the solution every hour.

Gelsemium 6c (phial)

Symptoms: The flu is characterized here by heaviness of the head, a red and congested face, heaviness of the eyelids, and absence of thirst. The sacrolumbar region is painful and the high temperature is accompanied by extreme weakness, leading to apathy, with shivering and trembling fits which are often violent.

Dosage: Dissolve 10 granules in a glass of water and give a dessertspoonful of the solution every hour.

N.B. Applying one or other of these two remedies to the young patient, according to the symptoms presented or ascertained, will be happily complemented by adding to the prepared solution a medicine designed to combat the attack of fever and its consequences (refer at this point to the chapter on fever).

The fresh remedy selected will be given in the same doses as previously, i.e., letting 10 granules of the antipyretic (fever-reducing) medication dissolve in the same glass of water as that which already contains one of the two constituents mentioned above.

NOSE-BLEEDS

A flow of red blood from the nose can be due to various causes, apart from blows received by the child in playground fights or knocks against a hard surface. Should this bleeding be repeated often, it is then indispensable to seek a medical opinion from the specialist.

However, in straightforward cases the mother will, as soon as the bleeding begins, be able to choose between two remedies, depending on the characteristics of the haemorrhage.

Melilotus 6c (phial)

Symptoms: The nose-bleed has been preceded by a significant redness of the face, a rush of blood to the head, and throbbing of the carotids (arteries). When the bleeding appears, it then relieves the little patient.

Dosage: 3 or 4 granules every 10-15 minutes.

Millefolium 3x (bottle)

Symptoms: Of bright-red blood, the nasal haemorrhage may be spontaneous or result from a blow or a fall on the face.

Dosage: 20 drops in half a glassful of water; give a teaspoonful every 10-15 minutes.

SORE THROATS

In children whose tonsils are habitually enlarged, the least chill risks the development of a defence reaction, which is more severe at this level, in the shape of acute inflammation of these lymphatic organs.

This inflammation then takes the form either of an ordinary sore throat or of tonsilitis with the appearance of purulent spots or pharyngeal exudates (throat discharges).

Two remedies are then to be applied, as the cause may be, while awaiting a medical opinion (if there is need of one).

Belladonna 6c (phial)

Symptoms: The throat is red and glossy, especially on the right. Swallowing is painful and the pain spreads to the ear. However, in spite of this impression of constriction of the pharynx, the little patient is thirsty and clamours for cold water. There may be a high temperature with the skin burning and moist with perspiration.

Dosage: Dissolve 10 granules in a glass of water and give a dessertspoonful of the solution every hour.

Mercurius solubilis 6c (phial)

Symptoms: In the case of this remedy, the sore throat, which is at first red, has a tendency, just like acute tonsillitis, to develop into suppuration. The tongue is swollen, coated with yellowish fur, and it retains the impress of the teeth. The young patient suffers from excessive salivation; the breath often smells; thirst is extreme and sweat copious, especially at night.

Dosage: Dissolve 10 granules in a glass of water and give a tablespoonful of the solution every hour.

N.B. In the case of tonsillitis, particularly if the temperature is up, it is worth mixing the two remedies indicated above in the proportion of 10 of each. Allow to dissolve in a glass of water and give a dessertspoonful every hour until the symptoms improve.

If the child is able to gargle, one will then advise putting 20 drops of *Phytolacca M.T.* (bottle) in half a bowl of boiled lukewarm water and gargling twice a day.

TONSILLITIS

Situated at the entrance to the upper respiratory tract, the tonsils, organs of lymphatic structure, must be considered as a protective barrier against the spread of infection to the level of that system.

When attacked acutely or chronically by invading microbes, the child's organism reacts by forming a very large number of lymphocytes (white blood cells) at the site of the organs which normally manufacture them, including the tonsils, which then enlarge in volume.

When the reaction assumes an acute, violent character accompanied by a high temperature, tonsillitis then takes the form of the sore throat whose first-aid treatment is indicated under the corresponding heading (see **SORE THROATS**). But if it is a matter of the existence of enlarged tonsils (and it is not always necessary to have them taken out), there will be a choice, according to the signs, between two remedies.

Baryta carbonica 6c (phial)

Symptoms: Chronic hypertrophy (enlargement) of the tonsils with tendency to repeated sore throats. This is complicated by the presence of painful ganglia (cystic swellings) at the level of the submaxillary (lower jaw) area.

Dosage: 3 granules three times a day between meals.

Silicea 6c (phial)

Symptoms: Increase in volume of the tonsil, particularly the left one, accompanied by a sensation of local pricking as though a needle were stuck into this organ. Swallowing is difficult and often painful. The child is very sensitive to cold and catches cold easily.

Dosage: 3 granules three times a day between meals

WHOOPING-COUGH

We shall give here only the homoeopathic treatment to be applied from the onset of this spasmodic affliction. Later on, Hahnemann remedies judiciously selected by the practitioner will appreciably curtail the development of the illness, which is often greatly drawn-out, and will protect the child from the complications which are always possible.

Coccus cacti 6c (phial)

Symptoms: The fit of whooping-cough, which occurs especially at night and wakens the little patient, ends with the expulsion of slimy and thick mucus, which hangs from each side of the mouth.

Dosage: Dissolve 10 granules in a glass of water and give a dessertspoonful of the solution every hour.

Drosera 6c (phial)

Symptoms: The cough is dry, racking, barking, and the fits of coughing follow one another so rapidly that the young patient has difficulty in drawing breath again in between them. The child stays restless and he complains of always being cold, even in bed.

Dosage: Dissolve 10 granules in a glass of water and give a dessertspoonful of the solution every hour.

Pertussinum 6c (dose)

Prepared from mucus of whooping-cough patients, this homoeopathic biotherapeutic is worth using both as a prophylactic in an infected environment and as a curative agent during the development of the illness.

Dosage: Prophylactically, give a single dose once a week, in the evening on retiring.

Curatively, in association with the remedies indicated above in accordance with the symptoms, give one dose twice a week on retiring.

2. DIGESTIVE ORGANS

APHTHAE (TINY ULCERS)

This surface lesion often attacks the mucous membranes of the mouth and gums. The paediatrician you consult will throw light on the many causes which can be at the root of these manifestations.

While waiting for his opinion, you will give first thought to relieving the local irritation.

Borax 6c (phial)

Symptoms: Presence of burning vesicles on the tongue and inner surface of the cheeks; the baby cries as soon as he wants to suck, yet he refuses the breast.

Dosage: Dissolve 10 granules in a glass of water and give a teaspoonful of the solution every half-hour.

Calendula M.T. (bottle)

Recommended also are two mouth washes per day with 20 drops of this mother tincture put into half a glassful of boiled lukewarm water.

APPETITE (Lack of)

It is not uncommon for the child to refuse even well-prepared food; the mother then gets rightly worried and seeks advice.

Depending on the complementary symptoms presented by the child, the choice will lie between two remedies.

Avena sativa 1x (bottle)

Symptoms: Lack of appetite after a serious or prolonged illness; general fatigue with sleeplessness.

Dosage: Give 20 drops in a little water before the two main meals.

Lycopodium 6c (phial)

Symptoms: This remedy suits the child with an hepatic (liver related) heredity. He constantly experiences voracious hunger, but – and this is the remedy's important characteristic which will govern its choice – this sensation of hunger is very quickly satisfied, for, no matter how little he has absorbed, he feels a sense of fullness in stomach and abdomen.

Dosage: 3 granules three times a day between meals.

CONSTIPATION

It is true that many laxatives can be given to the child whose motions are few and excretion difficult, but it is then necessary to avoid the abuse of them and, moreover, discover the true cause of the trouble. This latter task will devolve on the doctor consulted in the matter. For the young subject and in straightforward and occasional cases, there will be a choice between two remedies.

Alumina 6c (phial)

Symptoms: The stools are hard and their evacuation, already difficult, is in addition painful, even if the stools are soft; besides, for most of the time the child experiences no desire to empty his bowels.

Dosage: 3 granules three times a day between meals.

Taraxacum 1x (bottle)

Symptoms: Constipation with a mediocre appetite in the young hepatic subject; the child experiences a sensation of abdominal fullness. An important indication for this remedy is the nature of the tongue, which is like a 'map of the world,' i.e., covered with a whitish fur which scales off to give place to dark-red and sensitive patches.

Dosage: 20 drops in a little water before the two main meals.

DIARRHOEA (Attacks of)

The possibility of the appearance of frequent liquid stools in the child may admit of various causes. of which only three will be borne in mind here. They are among the commonest and can be arrested by the application of one of the medications examined below. As always, their choice will rest on the symptoms ascertained or experienced.

However, in the quite young child who is troubled by the persistence of this symptom, it is particularly important to have the doctor who is consulted arrange a more active treatment. The purpose of this is to mitigate the appearance of more serious disorders, in particular dehydration of the tissues and cholera-type symptoms.

Aethusa cynapium 6c (phial)

Symptoms: This remedy is indicated for the child who suffers from inability to tolerate milk, which is vomited as soon as it is ingested. The motions are watery, greenish, thick, preceded by stomach pains, and followed by a state of weakness with drowsiness. There may be a feverish condition with cold sweats. Worth noting are an absence of thirst and a need to be warmly covered up.

Dosage: Dissolve 10 granules in a glass of water and give a tablespoonful of the solution every half-hour.

Arsenicum album 6c (phial)

Symptoms: The diarrhoea, which usually comes on following

the consumption of watery fruit or tainted food, is characterized by evacuation of scalding, putrid stools, which are complicated by vomiting immediately after eating or drinking. The little patient is prostrated and thirsty for small amounts of water, which are, however, immediately thrown up.

Dosage: Dissolve 10 granules in a glass of water and give a dessertspoonful of the solution every hour.

Dulcamara 6c (phial)

Symptoms: In this case, the diarrhoea occurs after catching cold in damp weather or after resting or lying on damp ground. Hence it is the young camper's remedy. The diarrhoea is met with particularly in summer and autumn. The stools are yellow and watery and their evacuation is always preceded by pains in the abdomen and around the navel.

Dosage: Dissolve 10 granules in a glass of water and take a dessertspoonful of the solution every hour.

ENTERITIS

According to the symptoms presented or experienced, you will consult the headings **INTESTINAL COLIC** or **DIARRHOEA (Attacks of)**

HICCUPS

This minor reflex manifestation of digestive origin is, however, often distressing. It is due to a sharp contraction of the diaphragm, generally having as its cause an excess amount of air in the child's stomach.

Two remedies, always selected according to the symptomatology, will rapidly reduce these spasms.

Argentum nitricum 6c (phial)

Symptoms: The noisy and repeated flatulence comes on immediately after eating. The child who suffers from it experiences a violent desire for sweet things. He is usually in a perpetual state of excitement.

Dosage: 3 granules every 15-20 minutes.

Stramonium 6c (phial)

Symptoms: This remedy is indicated when there exists in the young person a spasmodic constriction of the oesophagus (gullet), preventing any swallowing, hence his rejection of all liquids.

Dosage: 3 granules every 30 minutes.

INDIGESTION

This indisposition, which is often commonplace, can take various forms, of which certain pathological expressions are examined in the earlier section dealing with diarrhoea and the one below on colic.

Here we shall look at only the gastric form of this digestive disorder, coming on after too big a meal or one consumed too quickly.

Nux vomica 6c (phial)

Symptoms: Sensation of a heavy weight in the stomach occurring an hour after eating and accompanied by distension. The little patient tries his best to vomit, but it is only with difficulty that he manages to bring up what he has just eaten. The abdomen is taut, swollen, and painful.

Dosage: 3 granules 3 or 4 times a day.

INTESTINAL COLIC

Independently of reactions of the appendix in young people predisposed to them, indigestion and chills on the stomach are usually the main causes of this sign.

Apart from diet and hot applications to the stomach (except. in the event of inflammation of the appendix, which contrariwise calls for ice), one will recommend a remedy whose symptomatology coincides with the clinical signs presented.

Colocynthis 6c (phial)

Symptoms: Cramp-type abdominal pains coming in paroxysms and forcing the young patient to bend double; this relieves him momentarily. Expelling stomach gas does not soothe him. The motions may be like those of dysentery and they are passed every time the youngster eats or drinks.

Dosage: Dissolve 10 granules in a glass of water and give a tablespoonful of the solution every half-hour.

INTESTINAL PARASITES

The child is often a carrier of intestinal worms whose presence is at the root of many pathological symptoms; these are often worrying for the mother. They include abnormal fatigue on the part of the child, extreme nervousness, and personality disorders, to cite only the main indications of this complaint.

In the face of these symptoms, a medical examination is imperative as well as an examination of the stools.

Depending upon the type of parasites shown to be present, the mother will be able to give the little patient one of the following three remedies.

Cina 6c (phial)

Symptoms: The young patient, who is, incidentally, irritable, temperamental, and trying, constantly rubs his nose. In addition, the presence of bluish circles is noted round eyes and mouth. At night, his sleep is disturbed and he grinds his teeth. He is apt to wake up frightened. The presence of roundworms or threadworms is noted in the stools.

Dosage: 3 granules four times a day between meals.

Taenifuge R.C.

A specific for the exclusive treatment of Taenia (tapeworm). Not a homoeopathic remedy, but one cannot speak of intestinal infestation with parasites without mentioning Taenia.

Tolerance of this medicine is perfect and it is absolutely harmless.

Dosage: For the child under 10, give a daily dose of 1 pill for each year of the child's age; over 10, give 10 pills a day.

Vermifuge L.H.F. (bottle)

By its composition, this homoeopathic compound not only acts on the symptomatology peculiar to parasitoses, but also contributes to altering the pathological basis, hence to avoiding the tendency of the undesirable visitors to multiply in the intestine.

Dosage: Before the two main meals give 20 drops in a little water for a fortnight each month until the parasites disappear.

KETONAEMIA

The abnormal presence of acetone in the blood is evidence of liver insufficiency mainly connected with metabolism of fats. It is characterized by vomiting, which is often considerable, and breath which smells like pippin apples.

Independently of a radical therapy which the doctor will decide and the institution of an appropriate diet, a first-aid remedy will enable the attack to be quickly relieved.

Senna 6c (phial)

Symptoms: Breath that smells aromatic; attacks of nausea and vomiting with yellowish diarrhoea; presence of acetone in the urine.

Dosage: 2 granules every 15-20 minutes.

TEETHING TROUBLES

I do not wish to encroach upon the prerogatives and attentions of the stomatologist, who is more qualified than I to treat the child's teeth. However, as auxiliaries to dental treatment, two remedies may be suggested to the mother, depending on two possibilities which may arise, namely pain and delayed dentition (teething).

Chamomilla 6c (phial)

Symptoms: Toothache, which often comes on at night and is hard to bear, is made particularly worse by having hot drinks. Conversely, it is relieved by cold ones. Worth noting, too, is a peculiarity which is altogether special to this remedy: the child has one cheek red and hot, while the other remains pale and cold.

Dosage: 2 or 3 granules every 20-30 minutes.

Silicea 6c (phial)

Symptoms: This remedy is to be recommended for the poorly-developed child who is thin, rachitic, slow in walking and who suffers from parodontal (dental) disease.

Dosage: 3 granules three times a day between meals.

THRUSH

This complaint, which affects the mucous membranes of the mouth and gums, is due to a fungoid growth; it may be met with in the new-born.

While you are waiting, if need be, for a medical opinion, one remedy can be applied for combating this symptom, which represents a particular type of stomatitis.

Mercurius cyanatus 6c (phial)

Symptoms: The mucous membrane of the mouth is covered in places with a thick and greyish coating; the tongue is white and the breath smells.

Dosage: Dissolve 10 granules in a glass of water and give a tablespoonful of the solution every hour.

VOMITING (Attacks of)

The regurgitation of the stomach contents can have various causes, including *interalia* ketonaemia and indigestion; these have already been examined in the respective sections, to which I refer the mother.

Under this heading we shall keep in mind only the vomiting of infants.

Aethusa cynapium 6c (phial)

Symptoms: The baby shows complete intolerance of milk; no sooner is it ingested than it is vomited in the form of thick acid clots; this abrupt throwing-up is followed by weakness and drowsiness.

Dosage: Dissolve 10 granules in a glass of water and give a teaspoonful of the solution every hour.

3. NERVOUS SYSTEM

CONVULSIONS

In a youngster, the appearance of involuntary contractions of the limbs is calculated to alarm or frighten those around him. In fact, this sign may be an omen of the birth of a serious complaint, of which the doctor, called in urgently, will decide the cause.

While waiting for him to come, you will be advised to apply a remedy immediately.

Cicuta virosa 4c (phial)

Symptoms: Spasmodic contractions of the whole body with stiffness of the nape of the neck and numerous contortions. These symptoms are provoked by noise and touch. Worth noting is a dilation of the pupils, which are insensitive to light.

Dosage: Dissolve 10 granules in a glass of water and give a tablespoonful of the solution every half-hour.

NEUROTIC DISORDERS

It stands to reason that disorders which can affect the child's mentality and behaviour must not be neglected by the parents, especially if these signs tend to look persistent or disturbing. A psychologist's opinion will be useful in many cases.

However, it is necessary to avoid falling into the opposite extreme, the result of exaggeration and too much attention paid to infantile whims, which are often the act of spoilt or badly brought-up children. Even if it entails being considered a martinet, one cannot deny that a good telling-off is frequently shown to be the best of remedies. But to dwell on this subject at any greater length would go far beyond the limits which we have set ourselves in compiling this work, which intends to remain essentially practical.

As far as we are concerned, therefore, we shall content ourselves with suggesting, under this heading, some homoeopathic remedies which can be given for certain psychological reactions; these can be considered as normal although they represent a definite handicap for the child and a source of concern for the parents.

Impatience (Tendency to)

Borax 6c (phial)

Symptoms: The child amenable to this remedy is anxious, irritable, and hypersensitive; he jumps at the least sound, screams and protests if one tips him forward to nurse him or put him down.

Dosage: 3 granules three or four times a day.

Thunderstorms (Fear of)

Rhododendron 4c (phial)

Symptoms: The youngster's sensitiveness becomes hard for him to bear when the electric charge in the atmosphere is too high, that is, prior to the thunderstorm which he dreads. Thus the child has a morbid dread of this phenomenon and he is particularly afraid of the sound of thunder.

Dosage: Give 3 granules every half-hour as soon as a storm threatens.

Violence (Tendency to)

Stramonium 6c (phial)

Symptoms: This remedy acts selectively on the nervous system, in particular on the brain substance, and it is indicated in cases of violent and random excitement; to be noted, too, in extreme cases is the impulse to strike, bite, and tear.

Dosage: 3 granules three or four times a day between meals.

Whims (Tendencies to)

Chamomilla 6c (phial)

Symptoms: This is the remedy for the child who is sensitive in the extreme, cross, and unable to tolerate a look or a word directed to him. Never satisfied, he wants a thing but, as soon as he is given it, rejects it and clamours for something else. He is, moreover, a restless, impatient child who will remain quiet only if nursed or taken out in the pram.

Dosage: 3 granules three or four times a day between meals.

N.B. To complete this brief survey devoted to certain neurotic disorders of childhood, we have reserved a special chapter for the psychological problems which chance to appear during school-days.

On this subject, therefore, we refer the mother to the fourth part of this work, entitled 'THE CHILD AT SCHOOL.'

SLEEP (Disturbances of)

For the child, sleep represents the most valuable token of good physical health and sound mental balance; hence it is important that this phase of rest and recovery should be respected and fully attended to.

The disturbances which may upset this normal physiological phase can admit of many causes, both physical and mental, which it will be the task of the doctor consulted for this purpose to bring to light and treat according to the recognized aetiology. Insomnia is a condition which is becoming more and more widespread, even in childhood, and for us it is naturally not a matter of giving the young insomniac sleeping-tablets, which are sources of poisoning, made even worse by the risk of habituation, hence of overdosage.

We have simply selected from the arsenal of homoeopathic medicines certain common remedies which lend themselves to being used in accordance with the type of insomnia or to alleviate the abnormal symptoms which threaten to lead to restless sleep.

Bed-wetting

Plantago 3x (bottle)

Symptoms: The child cannot hold back his water in the night and soaks his bed.

Dosage: 10-15 drops to be put in half a glass of water and taken half an hour before bedtime.

Grating the teeth

Cina 6c (phial)

Symptoms: During the night the child, who generally sleeps on his tummy, grinds his teeth. He is disturbed by violent jumps; he utters cries and wakes up in fright. These nervous symptoms are often associated with the presence of intestinal parasites, particularly threadwords.

Dosage: 5 granules one hour before bedtime.

Insomnia

Coffea 3x (bottle)

Symptoms: The child sleeps peacefully until the middle of the night, then he abruptly wakes up excited and asking to play.

Dosage: 10-15 drops in half a glass of water to be taken in sips.

Nightmares

Chamomilla 6c (phial)

Symptoms: While asleep the child who is a prey to nightmares cries and screams; he is anxious and often sleeps with his eyes wide open.

Dosage: 4 or 5 granules one hour before bedtime.

Restlessness

Ignatia 6c (phial)

Symptoms: Sleep is light and, while dropping off, the child is afflicted with convulsive movements of the limbs; this type of insomnia may come on following minor upsets or worries.

Dosage: 4 or 5 granules an hour before bedtime.

SLEEP-WALKING

Silicea 6c (phial)

Symptoms: This remedy is indicated for physically weak children whose defects of assimilation lead to arrested development; their sleep is broken and they are apt to get up in the night, walk in their sleep, and then go back to bed again.

Dosage: 3 granules three times a day between meals.

4. SKIN AND APPENDAGES

It has been said with good reason that the skin is the mirror of health. This tegument (membrane) covering the human body somehow reflects the subject's biological condition. Its outward appearance, colour, temperature, humidity, and dryness change with the pathological symptoms which affect the patient. Knowledge and clinical interpretation of these changes enable a diagnosis to be made in many cases by someone who knows how to observe them.

We recall these ideas only as a reminder and, above all, to make you properly understand the importance which must be given to cutaneous signs.

The same will apply, moreover, as far as the appendages are concerned, i.e., the hair and nails, which can also be damaged or marked by disease.

In the chapter which we now devote to this system and its ancillaries, we shall look at only the commonest occurrences, which do not always call for an authoritative medical opinion.

BLEPHARITIS

Inflammation of the eyelids can be due to a simple lack of cleanliness of the hands and, as a result, necessitates stricter attention to local hygiene.

If the complaint recurs – and in this case it is worth consulting the paediatrician – the blame may, in fact, be laid at the door of a rachitic condition affecting the little patient. This is particularly so if, at the same time, he shows an enlargement of the lymphatic glands of the neck or groins. As first-aid treatment while awaiting a medical opinion, recourse is to be had to a remedy which is particularly active in this complaint.

Euphrasia 6c (phial)

Symptoms: The eyelids are puffed, hot to the touch, and stuck together on waking in the morning. The eyes run and the watering is an irritant. To be noted, too, is the fact that the child shows some hypersensitiveness to light.

Dosage: 2 granules every hour.

N.B. In addition to this internal treatment, the mother is advised to bathe the youngster's eyelids with a pad of cotton wool soaked in an infusion of camomile or cornflower.

BOILS

To prevent inflammation of the hair-root produced by the staphylococcus from becoming an abcess, there will be a choice between two remedies in cases where the boils are of small dimensions.

Hepar sulphur 6c (phial)

Symptoms: Unhealthy skin of the young subject in whom every abrasion, even a small one, tends to suppurate. The pain of local drawing is soothed by applications of heat. If the pus runs, it smells like stale cheese and is often mixed with blood.

Dosage: 3 granules three or four times a day between meals.

Myristica sebifera 6c (phial)

Symptoms: This remedy hastens the formation of the core and leads to the bursting of the purulent pocket; hence its action can be compared to that of the lancet without any of its drawbacks.

Dosage: 3 granules three or four times a day between meals.

N.B. Before the boil breaks, *Cyrtopodium ointment* is to be applied locally; afterwards, to speed up healing, this can be replaced by *K.L.C. salve.*

BRUISES

There are several degrees of severity in the results of a knock sustained or a fall. It is always useful to ask for a medical opinion to disclose the possible existence of a more serious internal lesion.

Meanwhile, in straightforward cases, recourse is to be had to a specific remedy.

Bellis perennis 3x (bottle)

Symptoms: After a knock, the child feels tired and asks to stay in bed. The affected area is sensitive or painful and it shows discoloured patches which cannot be touched without arousing some sensitivity.

Dosage: 10-15 drops in a glass of water, one teaspoonful of which is to be given every half-hour.

N.B. Locally, on the area of bruising, apply hot, wet compresses impregnated with 20 drops of *Calendula M.T.*

BURNS

In this section we shall look only at cases of burns which do not involve serious consequences.

Two aspects of this accidental occurrence will be examined under the headings of simple burns without cutaneous vesicular reaction (blisters); and burns with blisters.

Care will be taken, however, not to forget that the severity of a burn depends not only on the depth of the lesion but also on its extent.

Simple burns

Independently of the local treatment and always in accordance with the symptoms presented, the mother will have a choice between two medicines.

Apis mellifica 6c (phial)

Symptoms: The part of the skin affected by the burn is slightly puffed without there being any blister formation; it is the site of acute, smarting pains which are improved by ice-packs.

Dosage: 3 granules every two or three hours.

Urtica urens 3x (bottle) *Symptoms*: In this case the burn is superficial and accompanied by itching reminiscent of that caused by nettle stings.

Dosage: Put 20 drops in a glass of water and give a teaspoonful of the solution every half-hour.

Burns with blisters

Cantharis 6c (phial)

Symptoms: The burn is caused by a boiling liquid; the skin is the site of an eruption of pruriginous (itchy) and fiery vesicles; cold applications help to soothe these pains.

Dosage: Dissolve 10 granules in a glass of water; give a teaspoonful every half-hour.

Rhus toxicodendron 6c (phial)

Symptoms: The skin affected is red and swollen with fiery blisters present, but, contrary to the previous remedy, cold applications make the painful sensation even worse whereas the latter will rather be soothed by heat.

Dosage: Dissolve 10 granules in a glass of water; give a teaspoonful every half-hour.

N.B. In both cases *Calendula ointment* is to be applied locally and the area of skin affected should be kept from exposure to the air by an adhesive dressing.

CHILBLAINS

This inflamed lesion, which attacks the extremities in particular, is caused by cold; but in children it indicates certain vitamin deficiencies, particularly vitamin D.

The aetiological factors having been determined, if necessary, by the doctor, the mother will be well advised to adopt a homoeopathic remedy which in this case is clearly indicated.

Agaricus 6c (phial)

Symptoms: Red and swollen, the extremities attacked are the site of sensations of burning and itching as if they had been stabbed by thousands of icicles.

Dosage: 3 granules three times a day between meals.

IMPETIGO

Of streptococcic or staphylococcic origin, this skin complaint is very contagious for the child who attends school. It shows itself by the appearance of pustules which dry up and then form thick, yellowish crusts.

Two remedies, always chosen according to the symptoms, will be used in this case.

Antimonium crudum 6c (phial)

Symptoms: The child, who is generally plump and regularly bad-tempered, presents skin vesicles which ooze and feel fiery and itchy, especially at night. The crusts which come away are thick and hard and have the colour of honey.

Dosage: 3 granules three or four times a day between meals.

Mezereum 6c (phial)

Symptoms: In this case, inflammation of the skin is complicated by ulcerations with the appearance of a purulent secretion covered by yellowish crusts. The vesicles which surround the affected area are fiery and pruriginous (itchy).

Dosage: 3 granules three or four times a day between meals.

INFANTILE ECZEMA

Independently of the consultant paediatrician's pinpointing a more appropriate diet, the mother will have a choice, according to the symptoms noted or experienced, between two remedies. On no account must antibiotics be given or ointments applied as these only help to make the complaint recur.

In fact, this skin symptom can be considered as a means of elimination of organic toxins; hence it is salutary. I have explained this at greater length in the section devoted to the significance of disease.

Berberis 6c (phial)

Symptoms: The 'dry' type of eczema particularly attacks the backs of the hands and the buttocks. The child experiences burning and itching sensations which are aggravated by scratching but improved by local cold compresses.

Dosage: 3 granules three or four times a day between meals.

Petroleum 6c (phial)

Symptoms: The 'weeping' type of eczema shows itself by the presence of small fiery and pruriginous (itchy) vesicles, especially at night; these ooze a watery fluid which then forms yellowish crusts.

Dosage: 3 granules three or four times a day between meals.

INSECT BITES AND STINGS

During the summer, the child who plays in the fields or meadows is often the victim of bee and wasp stings or bites from harvest-bugs. A remedy must be applied immediately, especially if the sting involves the mouth or throat, as it is known that consequences can be dramatic.

Apis mellifica 6c (phial)

Symptoms: Sudden swelling of the skin and mucous membranes at the site of the sting with burning pains; oedema (swelling) of the uvula and glottis with a feeling of suffocation.

Dosage: 3 granules every 15 minutes.

N.B. In addition to this internal treatment, if the sting involves the outer surface of the skin, dab locally with *Calendula M.T.* (bottle) at the rate of 10 drops on a sterile compress. If the sting involves the surface of the throat, immediately pour about twenty drops of this same remedy into the young patient's mouth.

MILK SPOTS (*See* IMPETIGO)

NAILS

The horny part which covers the upper surface of the extremity of the fingers can be the site of certain changes of colour or structure. They are often of definite diagnostic value if one will only pay some attention to them.

For children, we shall bear in mind here only four types of clinical expression. These concern the nail's nutrition itself (white spots, brittle nails), or its infection (in the form of whitlows), or the compulsion to bite the nails, which is so often encountered in childhood.

White spots

One of the most important causes of the existence of whitish ridges on the surface of the nail is represented by loss of calcium from the youthful organism. The sign can also be seen to appear after an infectious illness.

A remedy to increase calcium is recommended. It is *Osteocynesin L.H.F.* (box of tablets).

Dosage: 2 or 3 tablets before the two main meals.

Brittle nails

One can only repeat here what has been said in the previous section about the causes of this manifestation and its treatment.

Nail-biting

The medical term for a compulsion to bite one's nails is onychophagy.

In many cases, this symptom can be grouped with children's neurotic disorders, and it is then amenable to psychotherapy.

However, to assist the specialist in his task, a remedy will be recommended which applies particularly to the child's mentality and which will speed up the cure of this weakness

Baryta carbonica 6c (phial)

Symptoms: The child to whom this remedy applies is, on the whole, physically and mentally retarded. He is slow to understand, slow to retain. Worth noting from the physical viewpoint is the existence of chronically enlarged tonsils and extreme sensitivity to cold.

Dosage: 3 granules 3 or 4 times a day between meals.

Whitlow

Inflammation in the region of the nail is amenable to the same treatment as that which has been indicated for **BOILS** (see this term).

NAPPY RASH

The infant who is kept in prolonged contact with wet or soiled nappies may develop a skin eruption on the buttocks.

Apart from attention to local cleanliness, the following treatment is recommended to the mother.

Arsenicum album 6c (phial)

Symptoms: The skin is red, burning hot, and scaly; little flakes of skin are easily shed from the epidermis.

Dosage: Dissolve 10 granules in a glass of water and give a teaspoonful every hour.

N.B. Dust the inflamed area locally with *K.L.C. Powder*.

STYES

A stye is a small inflammation situated on the edge of the eyelid and may have a tendency to recur.

A homoeopathic treatment easily and swiftly puts an end to it.

Staphysagria 6c (phial)

Symptoms: The inner corner of the eyelid is the seat of a pruriginous (itchy) flare-up with the formation of a small abscess.

Dosage: 3 granules every three hours.

N.B. Twice a day bathe the affected eye with a cornflower infusion.

VULVOVAGINITIS

Ordinary local attention to cleanliness and hygiene puts an end to this inflammation of the external genitals; to hasten the cure an appropriate remedy is recommended to supplement it.

Hydrastis 6c (phial)

Symptoms: Itching of the vulva with an irritant and sticky discharge.

Dosage: 3 granules three times a day between meals.

WARTS

These little non-malignant growths on the skin are due to a proliferation of the papillae of the underlying dermal (deep skin) layer. They affect the face and hands in particular.

Depending on the character of the wart, there will be a choice between two remedies.

Thuja 6c (phial)

Symptoms: The wart, which is of average size, is hot and moist; it itches and bleeds easily.

Dosage: 3 granules twice a day between meals.

Nitric acid 6c (phial)

Symptoms: The wart, which is localized particularly on the back of the hand, is big, serrated, has a stalk, and oozes; further, it tends to bleed when one is getting washed.

Dosage: 3 granules three times a day between meals.

N.B. Apply locally twice a day a few drops of *Thuja M.T.* (bottle) on the wart.

5. FEVER AND FEVERS WITH RASH

Any abnormal raising of the body temperature, although measured on the thermometer, will have been appraised and expressed by a whole range of minor signs. They are bound to worry a mother, but should not alarm her excessively.

It must not be forgotten, in fact, that this symptom (as we have already explained in an earlier chapter) should be considered as the economy's means of defence against an invasion of microbes. In other words, it is a mechanism of organic purification, and the sturdier the child, the more violent the reactions are.

Indeed, the temperature must be maintained within reasonable limits so as to alleviate the drawbacks inherent in a long-standing hyperthermia (high fever), which may, moreover, be the initial sign of a more serious affliction.

Some homoeopathic remedies, which must always be selected in accordance with the established characteristics (to be examined in this chapter), will quite quickly bring the young patient relief from bouts of fever.

Of course, where the clinical phenomena persist in spite of the treatment applied, there is every reason to seek a medical opinion, for the causes of sudden rises of temperature are multiplied and may often pass unnoticed by the mother and those around her.

Under this heading, too, we have though it as well to give the initial therapy of ordinary fevers with rash, which are so common in childhood and which also have to be considered as so many attempts at organic purification.

FEVER

Faced with any sudden onset of fever and even before having uncovered its true cause, one will have a choice of two remedies, according to the signs which the youngster shows or presents.

Having recourse to traditional antipyretics (fever-reducing

agents) and to antibiotics, which are often poorly tolerated and inappropriately given, will thus be avoided.

Aconite 6c (phial)

Symptoms: The fever usually comes on after the child has been exposed to dry, cold conditions or a northerly wind. Thus it is a winter remedy. The face is red, the skin fiery and dry. The child is restless and shivers at the least movement. He is, in addition, thirsty and begs for lots of cold water. Lastly, the pulse is rapid and firm.

Dosage: Dissolve 10 granules in a glass of water and give a dessertspoonful of the solution every hour.

Belladonna 4c (phial)

Symptoms: The indications for this remedy rest on the following signs: the child is in low spirits; the skin is burning and throws off heat; but, unlike the previous case, it is moist on account of profuse sweating; the febrile condition may, in some cases, lead to delirium; lastly, note the absence of thirst.

Dosage: Dissolve 10 granules in a glass of water and give a dessertspoonful of the solution every hour.

FEVERS WITH RASH

In this manual we don't claim to give the exhaustive treatment of all the fevers with rash with which the child may be afflicted. In their entirety, they can be considered as so many defence reactions of the young subject to hereditary pathological traits. Their diagnosis and treatment will depend, in the majority of cases, on the paediatrician.

However, from the start of minor symptoms which can make the mother anxious, from the appearance of this or that eruption or this or that symptom, especially if they arise in a contagious environment, recourse will be had to a few simple remedies (which in the end are the most effective) pending the arrival of the doctor.

MEASLES

This contagious illness is characterized by an eruption of small red spots on the surface of the skin.

As soon as the first symptoms appear, the mother will have recourse to two first-aid remedies.

Aconite 6c (phial)

Symptoms: The skin is burning hot; it is the site of an

erythematous (inflammatory) eruption leaving areas of healthy skin. The fever is signalled by shivering and the child is restless, often distressed too. He is thirsty for lots of cold water.

Dosage: Dissolve 10 granules in a glass of water and give a dessertspoonful of the solution every hour.

Euphrasia 6c (phial)

Symptoms: This remedy is indicated as soon as the child shows constant and irritant watering of the eyes; his eyelids are puffy and hot; there may also be a watery nasal discharge.

Dosage: Dissolve 10 granules in a glass of water and give a dessertspoonful of the solution every hour.

N.B. In a contagious environment and even before any sign of eruption, give the child a single dose of *Morbillinum 6c* (dose) as a preventive measure at bedtime.

MUMPS

Also contagious, this illness is linked with the activity of a virus. It shows itself as a sudden acute inflammation of the parotid (beside the ear) glands, which enlarge and so give the child a typical facial outline.

As in the previous case, two remedies must be applied immediately the early signs appear.

Belladonna 4c (phial)

Symptoms: Painful swelling of the parotids; the skin of the face is burning and glossy; the temperature is up and the child is listless.

Dosage: Dissolve 10 granules in a glass of water and give a dessertspoonful of the solution every hour.

Mercurious solubilis 6c (phial)

Symptoms: Painful swelling of the parotids; the little patient produces a lot of saliva and the tongue, which is swollen, holds the imprint of the teeth; profuse sweating brings no relief.

Dosage: Dissolve 10 granules in a glass of water and give a dessertspoonful of the solution every hour.

SCARLET FEVER

This feverish illnes of microbial origin can have serious complications as regards the ears in the shape of otitis, or as regards the kidneys in the shape of acute nephritis; hence it must naturally be looked after by the doctor.

But, pending his opinion and as soon as suspicious signs of a sore throat appear, especially in a contagious environment, recourse will immediately be had to the remedies indicated for that complaint. (See the heading **SORE THROATS**.)

VARICELLA (Chicken-pox)

This eruption, which is of a virus nature and contagious, is characterized initially by the appearance of red spots. These are soon followed by vesicles which disappear at the end of about ten days.

The mother will have recourse to two remedies shortening the period of development of this illness which, furthermore, does not involve any degree of severity.

Belladonna 6c (phial)

Symptoms: This is the remedy to be applied right from the initial stage of the illness. The skin is red with erythematous (inflammatory) patches, the eruption appearing suddenly.

Dosage: Dissolve 10 granules in a glass of water and give a dessertspoonful of the solution every hour.

Rhus toxicodendron 6c (phial)

Symptoms: This is the remedy for the next stage: eruptions of vesicles which burn and itch, causing the child to scratch.

Dosage: 3 granules every other hour during the day.

6. GENERAL CONDITION

In this section and under this title, I thought it as well to class some of the minor complaints or certain pathological aspects not of major severity which have been unable to find a place within the compass of the illnesses examined in the previous chapters.

I am concerned here only with symptoms likely to affect the child's general condition or to represent the clinical expression of a more serious illness, which in any case will call for a medical opinion.

Throughout this survey I have suggested to the mother only some homoeopathic remedies which, in certain cases, will be enough to bring a rapid lessening of the symptoms confirmed or experienced by the young patient. Or again taking them will, if need be, permit of the initiation of a more complete therapy which will then be given by the paediatrician consulted in this connection.

ANAEMIA IN THE INFANT

Lack of iron in the food intake means a risk of creating a state of deficiency prejudicial to the health of the quite young child who is still limited to a milk diet.

It is advisable to consult the paediatrician to see to the details of a regime richer in iron.

One remedy will happily complete the readjustment of the recommended diet.

Iron, Gluconate of (ampoule)

Dosage: Give one ampoule per day dry under the tongue.

CONVALESCENCE (*See* FATIGUE)

DECREASE OF CALCIUM IN TEETH AND BONES

Diminution of the level of calcium in the child's organism finds expression in a whole range of symptoms, including *inter alia* fatigue, abnormal sensitivity to cold, and irritability. These are all signs which the paediatrician will interpret to arrange an appropriate treatment.

As for the mother, if she looks at her offspring's nails, she will note in cases of decrease of calcium the presence of white spots. Independently of a regime rich in calcium and mineral salts laid down by the doctor, the child will benefit by regular use of the following remedy.

Calcium compound 3c trituration (powder)

Dosage: Give two or three measures of the powder before the two main meals.

FATIGUE

This distressing feeling of lassitude overcomes the child in certain circumstances, such as physical over-exertion, stress at school, nervous tension, too rapid growth, sequelae of infectious illnesses, etc.

Where the condition persists, the mother will be wise to seek a medical opinion. I shall content myself with indicating here two remedies which, in all the above-mentioned cases and always according to the symptoms confirmed, will bring valuable help to the tired youngster.

Alfalfa 1x (bottle)

Symptoms: Heaviness of the head, especially at the level of the occipital (back of the head) region; poor appetite with excessive thirst, constant desire for sweets; broken sleep.

Dosage: Give 20 drops in a little water before the two main meals.

Avena sativa 1x (bottle)

Symptoms: Lack of general muscle tone with insomnia; nervous fatigue and debility following feverish illnesses; headaches with a burning sensation on the crown of the head, extending to the nape of the neck.

Dosage: Give 20 drops before the two main meals.

FONTANELLES (Delayed closure of)

These gaps situated between the bones of the skull are sometimes slow to knit in completing the growth of the baby's head.

With a view to speeding up the entire hardening of this part of the body, a combination of two homoeopathic remedies, one simple, the other compound, will be advised.

Silicea 6c (phial)

Symptoms: The child who is amenable to this remedy is thin and rachitic. (Suffering from rickets). He perspires easily from the head, which is increased in size, the fontanelles remaining open. This child, moreover, is slow in walking; he is irritable, headstrong; he jumps at the least noise.

Dosage: Give 3 granules three times a day.

Osteocynesin L.H.F. (tablets)

Dosage: Give 2 tablets before the two main meals.

GANGLIA

These swellings, situated along the course of the lymphatic vessels, are grouped at the level of the neck, groins, and abdomen.

Their increase in size, which can be felt and seen, is evidence of a defence reaction by the organism against an infectious condition, either hereditary or acquired.

Here I shall, of course, look at only the latent forms, which develop without an increase in temperature. In other types of cases, the appearance of a febrile ganglionic hypertrophy (overgrowth) will call for a medical opinion, for it may precede or accompany a more serious illness.

In straightforward cases, two remedies will (always according to the symptoms noted) be particularly indicated.

Drosera 6c (phial)

Symptoms: Increase in size of cervical (neck) or inguinal (groin) ganglia (nerve cells); frequent pains in the joints; irritating cough through tickling of the larynx as soon as the child is lying down.

Dosage: Give 3 granules three or four times a day between meals.

Sulphur iodatum 6c (phial)

Symptoms: The cervical adenopathy (neck swelling) is generally accompanied by chronic hypertrophy of the tonsils; furthermore, there is a tendency to herpes (skin eruption) of the lips.

Dosage: Give 3 granules three or four times a day outside of mealtimes.

GROWTH (Disorders of)

The child's progressive development may be retarded or even give rise to certain so-called 'growing' pains at the level of the epiphyses[1].

The causes which lie at the root of one or other of these occurences can be many and often result from glandular disorders. The latter then call for the arranging of opotherapy[2] under the supervision of the doctor who has been consulted.

Pending this and according to the case seen, some homoeopathic remedies are particularly indicated.

Delayed growth

Depending on the symptoms noted, there will be a choice between two remedies.

Calcarea carbonica 6c (phial)

Symptoms: The child amenable to this remedy has a large stomach and a large head, which is often bathed in sweat at night; this perspiration has a sour smell and soaks the pillow.

[1] Plural of *epiphysis*, the spongy extremity of a bone. – *Trans.*

[2] Opotherapy: treatment by administration of extracts of animal organs. – *Trans.*

He is slow in learning to walk; his skin is chalky-white and his tonsils are enlarged.

Dosage: Give 3 granules three times a day.

Natrum muriaticum 6c (phial)

Symptoms: This remedy corresponds rather to a child who is thin with delayed development; he is habitually depressed, seeks solitude, readily sulks, and suffers from headaches characterized by violent throbbings as if the brain were being struck by hammer blows.

Dosage: Give 3 granules three times a day.

Growing pains

In this case, before a medical opinion if there is need of one, recourse will be had to a remedy which acts on the developing bone structure.

Calcarea phosphorica 6c (phial)

Symptoms: The pains in the bones are gnawing, gripping, and accompanied by a sensation of stiffness in the neck and muscles; further, these pains are made worse by cold and damp weather. As regards capacity for movement, the child cannot climb the stairs without complaining.

Dosage: Give 3 granules three times a day

INOCULATION (After-effects of)

At this point much could be said about inoculation's carried out to-day on a very large scale with the aim of avoiding the development of acute illnesses liable to afflict the child.

The present wholesale use of inoculation carries the risk of ultimately involving the recipients in serious after-effects. This especially applies to youthful organisms ill prepared to receive more or less toxic doses of foreign proteins.

Many authorities now admit, moreover, that inoculations no longer seem to be justified by modern science. However, ignorance of the law – and still less evasion of it – being no excuse, it is obligatory to have children subjected to a 'toxifying' of which one cannot always assess the dangers and know all the consequences.[1] It will be pointed out that the homoeopathic pharmacopoeia includes in its arsenal a series of

[1] The author is referring to France. Readers are reminded that inoculation is not compulsory in the United Kingdom. – *Trans*.

vaccines or '*nosodes*,' to use the recognized term, which can be administered orally and of which the prescription and dosage will be left to the judgement of the Hahnemann physician.

Whatever the circumstances, you will feel all the better for giving the child two remedies which, depending on the symptoms observed, will counteract the harmful effects of inoculation.

Silicea 6c (phial)

Symptoms: This remedy is particularly indicated for the rachitic (suffering from rickets) child who evinces attacks of asthma following repeated vaccinations.

Dosage: Give 3 granules four times a day for one week after the use of the vaccine.

Thuja 6c (phial)

Symptoms: The skin surface of the child amenable to this remedy often shows signs of warts. The nails are brittle and break easily. The existence of adenopathies (swellings) can be noted. Hence this remedy will be prescribed and used to forestall the ill effects of vaccinations.

Dosage: Give 3 granules four times a day for one week after the use of the vaccine.

IV
THE CHILD AT SCHOOL

INTRODUCTION

Separation, even for a moment, from the family circle can, in some sensitized children, bring about the birth of either physical or mental disturbances.

Moreover, one cannot help noticing a regular increase in the number of children who are abnormal or mentally handicapped or otherwise maladjusted to social life, as represented for the youngster by *inter alia* the school environment. The appearance of abnormal reactions is often linked with starting school, and in some cases there is a risk of their being prolonged throughout this period in the child's life.

Of course, as a corollary, the marks given by the teacher to the pupil show the effects of these reactions and often form the subject of demands or lack of understanding on the part of the family. Hence, the child being the first victim of this, it is at that stage when the doctor must intervene to try to restore order to the young scholar's state of mental health. Once again, our aim in the course of this essentially practical work is not to exhaust so vast and complex a subject as the detailed examination of the psycho-pathological or somatic signs which can change for the worse the physical and mental health of the child at school.

We shall bear in mind here only some of the commonest aspects of the above signs, considered solely from the angle of their homoeopathic treatment. In fact, the latter will, in each of the simple cases which have been looked at in the course of this part of our work, be capable of complementing happily and without risk of medicinal poisoning a psychological re-education carried out under the auspices and supervision of the relevant specialist.

SYMPTOMS

AGGRESSIVENESS

Under this term will be defined that psychological tendency which is expressed in the subject's state of hostility towards others.

Selected always in accordance with the observed symptoms, two remedies will help to restore to the child a measure of mental reduction of tension.

Hepar sulphur 6c (phial)

Symptoms: Irritation at the slightest cause in a child who is habitually peevish and sulky; impulse to do harm, to set fire.

Dosage: 3 granules three times a day between meals for three weeks in the month.

Lycopodium 6c (phial)

Symptoms: Extreme touchiness manifesting in sudden outbursts of anger and the use of strong language. To be noted here is the wizened look of the child, who often wakes up in the morning with a bad temper.

Dosage: 3 granules three times a day between meals for three weeks in the month.

ANXIETY

This feeling of physical anxiety is characterized by the occurrence of a burdensome sense of oppression, which at times is even painful. Depending on the symptoms observed in the child, there will be a choice between two remedies.

Arsenicum album 6c (phial)

Symptoms: In this case the anxiety is accompanied by extreme restlessness. The child is afraid to stay by himself and is unable to keep quiet. In the night he generally wakes up between 1 a.m. and 3 a.m. with an intolerable sense of anxiety.

Dosage: 3 granules three times a day between meals for three weeks in the month.

Aurum metallicum 6c (phial)

Symptoms: Here the sense of anxiety is complicated by a state of depression, which may go as far as disgust with life and thoughts of suicide in spite of the fear of death.

Dosage: 3 granules three times a day for three weeks in the month.

ATTENTION (Lack of)

Often the school-child undergoes some difficulty in focusing his mind on his work and his marks show the effects of it.

A so-called 'constitutional' remedy will enable him to overcome this handicap.

Calcarea carbonica 6c (phial)

Symptoms: The child is apathetic, slow in understanding, slow in complying, and mental work tires him out; to be also noted in him are sudden impulses to run or to jump out of the window.

Dosage: 3 granules three times a day between meals for three weeks in the month.

BACKWARDNESS AT SCHOOL

In the young child at school, a certain number of factors, as much physical as mental, may arise to bring about some lag in the normal progress of his education: a constitutional tendency, the aftermath of serious or prolonged illnesses, inability to assimilate the school curriculum, which is often too heavy and too full, emotional or family conflicts, etc.

For one or other of the causes indicated above and always in accordance with the symptoms noted or experienced, the therapeutic choice will turn to one of the two remedies proposed below.

Calcarea carbonica 6c (phial)

Symptoms: Here the backwardness develops in psychological ground with underlying anxiety; there ensues a certain slowness in understanding and execution, so much so that mental work tires the youngster and on that account he evades the task to be accomplished.

Dosage: 3 granules three times a day between meals for three weeks in the month.

Graphites 6c (phial)

Symptoms: This remedy is better suited to a child who is overweight, who feels the cold and is habitually listless; even minimal exertion discourages him and he is unable to concentrate his thoughts on any subject whatever; very sensitive, he cries for nothing.

Dosage: 3 granules three times a day between meals for three weeks in the month.

BRAIN FAG

Some other causes of fatigue have been dealt with in the section of this book devoted to the sick child. Independently of these, the child may, during his school year, experience a certain lassitude on account of the mental exertion required. It can be overcome thanks to the homoeopathic remedy indicated in this particular case.

Calcarea phosphorica 6c (phial)

Symptoms: Difficulty in carrying out brain work due to the occurrence of headaches; these may, moreover, be accompanied by attacks of diarrhoea.

Dosage: 3 granules three times a day between meals.

DYSLEXIA

The proportion of today's school-children troubled by this disability is 10 per cent. It finds expression in difficulty in learning to read resulting from the impossibility of identifying, understanding, and reproducing written symbols.

For instance, the child will confuse P and B, D and B; he may reverse or mix up letters, syllables, and words, or make mistakes in the order of sequence of letters.

Independently of remedial therapy under the supervision of a specialist, a homoeopathic remedy encourages a return to a more normal mental state.

Lycopodium 6c (phial)

Symptoms: Difficulty in finding the right word to express himself; the child confuses words and syllables and, when writing, forgets letters and words.

Dosage: 3 granules three times a day between meals for three weeks in the month.

INDECISION

In the school-child, the feeling of uncertainty and the impression of hesitating when faced with a decision to be taken are seen in difficulty in solving the problems that school life sets him – lessons to be learnt and exercises to be worked.

For this disability, which can only hold back the child's education, the following remedy is recommended.

Calcarea fluorica 6c (phial)

Symptoms: Here we are in the presence of a child who cannot make any decision from day to day even about the most trifling matters; there ensues a state of constant anxiety and depression.

Dosage: 3 granules three times a day between meals for three weeks in the month.

IRRITABILITY

A child of an habitually sensitive temperament is sometimes apt to respond to the emotional shocks of school life with an attitude which, although not overt aggressiveness (*see this term*), may be accompanied by blunt reactions. The consequences of this are often damaging to the normal course of schooling.

In this case you will have a choice between two homoeopathic remedies which, depending on the symptoms noted in the child, will bring him greater peace of mind.

Argentum nitricum 5c (phial)

Symptoms: This remedy is perfectly suited to the young person who is habitually restless, anxious, and in a rush, for whom time passes too slowly, and who would like a speedy end to what he wants to take on even before he has started it.

Dosage: 3 granules three times a day between meals for three weeks in the month.

Chamomilla 6c (phial)

Symptoms: Extreme touchiness with impatience; the child can't stand being contradicted and flies into a rage over a mere trifle. Worth noting, too, in the physical sphere, is an intolerance of pain which is out of all proportion to the cause inducing it.

Dosage: 3 granules three times a day between meals for three weeks in the month.

MEMORY (Lack of)

Difficulty in retaining what has been taught represents a genuine handicap for the young scholar. Many causes can be at the root of this psychological shortcoming, and it will often be up to the psychologist who is consulted to unearth them.

A remedy will, however, be recommended to help in the

retraining of this important brain function.

Phosphoric acid 3x (bottle)

Symptoms: Memory impairment in the school-child, who is exhausted by class work, with inability to link two ideas together and to find the right words to express himself.

Dosage: 10-15 drops in a little water before the two main meals.

STAGE-FRIGHT

The fear, often panic, which the school-child may experience either on reciting and demonstrating on the black-board in front of his class-mates or prior to examination papers, is fortunately combated by a highly specific and very effective homoeopathic remedy.

Gelsemium 6c (phial)

Symptoms: Morbid dread of speaking in front of an audience or even in front of a third person; this emotional attitude is accompanied by bouts of uncontrollable trembling and diarrhoea.

Dosage: 5 granules two or three times a day between meals.

V

CHILDREN'S REMEDIES

INTRODUCTION

In the final part of this work I aim to make the technique of homoeopathic prescribing even better understood. So I shall now give in the following pages the main symptoms peculiar to each of the remedies which have been indicated in the earlier pages. They will thus complement the individual symptoms of the conditions described and studied with reference to the selected medicine in the purely clinical part – all this in accordance with the signs observed in the child or experienced by him.

Once more, these remedies have been chosen according to the norm of the homoeopathic principle, i.e., according to the appearance and modalities of the clinical sign that has been ascertained. They will very easily enable you to compare them with those which you have been in a position to note in the young patient.

You will, therefore, observe the child and carefully detect the signs which he betrays or feels.

You will then refer to the clinical part for the remedies indicated in the section on the corresponding illness. You will compare the symptoms observed in the young subject with those given by that remedy which, according to your own findings and observations, appears to you best indicated by the case to be treated.

Such is the secret (if secret it is) of homoeopathic prescribing. As already said many times in the preceding pages, prescribing is based upon *observation* and the most exact *comparison* possible between the signs of the illness to be treated and the remedy to be applied.

MATERIA MEDICA

A

ACONITUM (Aconite)

Symptoms: Acute, unbearable ear-ache, especially at night, after a cold, dry spell; feverishness with shivering and restlessness; high temperature after exposure to dry, cold weather; thirst for lots of cold water; skin dry and burning and the site of a red rash.

Indications: **ACUTE OTITIS – FEVER – MEASLES.**

AETHUSA CYNAPIUM (Fool's-parsley)

Symptoms: Inability to take milk, which is vomited in thick clots; watery, greenish motions preceded by stomach pains and followed by debility with drowsiness.

Indications: **DIARRHOEA – VOMITING.**

AGARICUS MUSCARIUS (Amanita fly agaric)

Symptoms: Itching and burning sensation at the level of the extremities, which are red and swollen.

Indications: **CHILBLAINS.**

ALETRIS FARINOSA (Unicorn root, Colic root)

Symptoms: Heaviness in the lower part of the abdomen with false labour pains.

Indications: **TENDENCY TO MISCARRIAGE.**

ALFALFA (Lucerne)

Symptoms: Heaviness of the head, especially in the occipital region; poor appetite and excessive thirst; desire for sweets; broken sleep.

Indications: **FATIGUE.**

ALLIUM CEPA (Onion)

Symptoms: Frequent sneezing with a lot of watery nasal secretions irritating to the nostrils and upper lip.

Indications: **HEAD COLDS.**

ALUMINA (Clay)

Symptoms: Hard stools with pains on evacuation; persistent constipation with no desire to attend stool.

Indications: **CONSTIPATION.**

ANTIMONIUM CRUDUM (Black antimony sulphide)

Symptoms: Oozing blisters on the skin with a sensation of local burns and itches; formation of thick, hard scabs of the colour of honey.

Indications: **IMPETIGO.**

ANTIMONIUM TARTARICUM (Emetic)

Symptoms: Loose, spasmodic cough accompanied by a good deal of rattling in the throat; no expectoration; breathing heavy and difficult; with dilation of the nostrils.

Indications: **ACUTE BRONCHITIS – COUGHS.**

APIS MELLIFICA (Honey-bee)

Symptoms: Skin bloated with absence of lumps or blisters; partial or general swelling with albuminuria (protein in urine); stabbing and burning pains; absence of thirst; desire for cold milk.

Indications: **ALBUMINURIA – BURNS AND SCALDS – INSECT BITES AND STINGS.**

ARGENTUM NITRICUM (Nitrate of silver)

Symptoms: Restlessness with extreme anxiety; fear of remaining alone; waking up with a sense of anxiety between 1 a.m. and 3 a.m.; watery, burning nasal secretions which cause the skin to peel; fits of sneezing bring no relief; diarrhoea on eating watery fruit or tainted food; scalding, putrid motions with vomiting; skin red, burning, scaly.

Indications: **COLDS – DIARRHOEA – NAPPY RASH – ANXIETY.**

AURUM (Gold)

Symptoms: Anxiety with low spirits and disgust with life; suicidal tendency with fear of death.

Indications: **ANXIETY.**

AVENA SATIVA (Oats)

Symptoms: Nervous exhaustion with sleeplessness; lack of muscle tone; loss of appetite after a serious or lengthy illness.

Indications: **DECREASE OF CALCIUM IN TEETH AND BONES – LACK OF APPETITE.**

B

BARYTA CARBONICA (Barium carbonate)

Symptoms: Delayed mental and physical development; chronic overgrowth of the tonsils; tendency to sore throats; enlarged and painful submaxillary ganglia (cystic swellings in lower jaw region).

Indications: **TONSILLITIS – NAIL-BITING.**

BELLADONNA (Deadly nightshade)

Symptoms: Reddened, glossy-looking throat with pain on swallowing which extends to the ear; painful swelling of the parotid (beside the ear) glands; high temperature; skin fiery and moist with red patches; absence of thirst; tendency to delirium.

Indications: **ACUTE SORE THROAT – FEVER – MUMPS – CHICKEN POX.**

BELLIS PERENNIS (Daisy)

Symptoms: Black-and-blue spots painful to the touch; fatigue after a blow or a fall.

Indications: **BRUISES.**

BERBERIS (Barberry)

Symptoms: Pruriginous (itchy) skin eruptions with burning, aggravated by scratching and improved by cold compresses.

Indications: **INFANTILE ECZEMA.**

BORAX (Sodium borate)

Symptoms: Oversensitiveness with anxiety and inability to stand the least noise; burning vesicles (blisters) on the tongue and internal surface of the cheeks; refusal of the breast by the baby, who squalls as soon as he wants to suck.

Indications: **APHTHAE – IMPATIENCE.**

BRYONIA ALBA (White bryony)

Symptoms: Dry, erratic cough which gets worse at the slightest movement and is accompanied by acute pains in the chest.

Indications: **ACUTE BRONCHITIS – COUGHS.**

C

CALADIUM (Arum lily)

Symptoms: Depression and fatigue from abuse of tobacco; loss of memory; irritability at the least noise.

Indications: **ANTIDOTE FOR TOBACCO.**

CALCAREA CARBONICA (Oyster shell)

Symptoms: Slow in learning and walking; lack of attention; fatigue from mental work; backwardness at school; enlarged head; large abdomen; sour-smelling night sweats which soak the pillow; enlarged tonsils; chalky-white skin.

Indications: **DISORDERS OF GROWTH – BACKWARDNESS AT SCHOOL.**

CALCAREA FLUORICA (Calcium fluoride)

Symptoms: Impossibility of making a decision, even about the most trivial matters; anxiety state with depression.

Indications: **INDECISION.**

CALCAREA PHOSPHORICA (Calcium phosphate)

Symptoms: Difficulty in carrying out brain work; tendency to headaches; gnawing pains in the bones, tension with stiffness in the neck and muscles made worse by cold and damp weather; climbing stairs is painful.

Indications: **GROWING PAINS – BRAIN FAG.**

CALCIUM COMPOUND (Salts combined with calcium)

Indications: **DECREASE OF CALCIUM IN TEETH AND BONES.**

CALENDULA (Marigold)

Symptoms: External sores with or without loss of skin; antidote for bee or wasp stings.

Indications: **BURNS – BRUISES – SORES – INSECT BITES AND STINGS.**

CANTHARIS (Cantharides)

Symptoms: Occurrence of burning and pruriginous (itchy) blisters on the skin, alleviated by cold compresses.

Indications: **BURNS.**

CHAMOMILLA (Camomile)

Symptoms: Morbid irritability and constant dissatisfaction; restlessness and impatience; impossibility of tolerating opposition; anger over trifles; toothache at night relieved by cold drinks; one cheek red and hot, the other cold and pale; tears and screams during sleep; eyes wide open at night.

Indications: **TEETHING TROUBLES – IRRITABILITY – TENDENCY TO WHIMS – NIGHTMARES.**

CHINA (Quinine)

Symptoms: Sequelae of repeated or prolonged haemorrhages

with anaemia and drop in body temperature.
Indications: **HAEMORRHAGES.**
CICUTA VIROSA (Water hemlock, Cowbane)
Symptoms: Spasmodic contractions of the muscles of the body; stiffness of the nape of the neck; contortions.
Indications: **CONVULSIONS.**
CINA (Santonica, Worm-seed)
Symptoms: Irritability; capricious temper; dark rings around the eyes and mouth; itchy nose; insatiable hunger; jumps and grinds teeth during sleep.
Indications: **INSOMNIA – INTESTINAL PARASITES.**
COCCULUS (Cocculus indicus)
Symptoms: Nausea with dizziness and hiccups; empty feeling in the stomach; aversion to the smell of food.
Indications: **NAUSEA.**
COCCUS CACTI (Cochineal)
Symptoms: Fits of whooping-type coughing, especially at night, ending in the bringing up of thick mucus.
Indications: **WHOOPING-COUGH.**
COFFEA (Coffee)
Symptoms: Sudden waking in the middle of the night; the child cannot go to sleep again and asks to play.
Indications: **INSOMNIA.**
COLOCYNTHIS (Colocynth)
Symptoms: Cramplike, paroxysmal abdominal pains forcing the victim to bend double; dysentery-type stools after eating or drinking.
Indications: **INTESTINAL COLIC.**

D

DROSERA (Sundew)
Symptoms: Dry, racking, barking cough; successive fits of coughing so rapid that the patient can get his breath again only with difficulty; enlarged cervical (neck) or inguinal (groin) ganglia (nerve cells); pains in the joints.
Indications: **WHOOPING-COUGH – GANGLIA (SWELLING).**
DULCAMARA (Bitter-sweet, Woody nightshade)
Symptoms: Diarrhoea in humid weather occurring in summer

or autumn; watery and yellowish motions, the evacuation of which is preceded by abdominal pains.

Indications: **SEASONAL DIARRHOEA.**

E

EUPATORIUM (Feverwort, Thoroughwort, Boneset, Hemp agrimony)

Symptoms: General sensation of aching and stiffness in the bones and muscles; pains in the eyeballs; morning temperature up and accompanied by shivering.

Indications: **FLU.**

EUPHRASIA (Euphrasy, Eyebright)

Symptoms: Eyelids swollen, burning, and stuck together on waking; irritant watering of the eyes; sensitivity to light; watery discharge from the nose.

Indications: **BLEPHARITIS – MEASLES.**

F

FERRUM PHOSPHORICUM (Phosphate of iron)

Symptoms: Spasms of pain in the affected ear with throbbing, relieved by cold compresses; dry, spasmodic, painful cough; expectoration sometimes flecked with blood; high temperature with rapid and weak pulse.

Indications: **ACUTE BRONCHITIS – ACUTE OTITIS.**

G

GELSEMIUM (Yellow jasmine)

Symptoms: Morbid fear of speaking in public; tendency to fits of trembling and diarrhoea due to emotion; heaviness of the head and eyelids; face red and congested; backache; high temperature with extreme weakness accompanied by shivers and fits of trembling.

Indications: **FLU – STAGE FRIGHT.**

GRAPHITES (Graphite)

Symptoms: Constant apathy in an overweight child who feels the cold; tiredness at the least effort; incapable of concentrating; cries for nothing.

Indications: **BACKWARDNESS AT SCHOOL.**

H

HELONIAS DIOICA (Helonias)

Symptoms: Weakness and heaviness in the lower part of the pregnant woman's abdomen.

Indications: **ALBUMINURIA.**

HEPAR SULPHURIS (Liver-coloured sulphur compound)

Symptoms: Irritation at the slightest cause; impulse to do wrong; unhealthy skin; tendency for the slightest injury to suppurate; discharge of pus smelling like stale cheese.

Indications: **AGGRESSIVENESS – ANTIDOTE TO ANTIBIOTICS – FURUNCULOSIS.**

HYDRASTIS

Symptoms: Thick and yellowish mucous discharge; catarrhal condition with weakness and emaciation; itching of the vulva (external female genitals).

Indications: **HEREDITARY TAINTS – VULVO-VAGINITIS IN GIRLS.**

I

IGNATIA (St Ignatius's bean)

Symptoms: Attacks of migraine resulting from abuse of tobacco with the 'nail driven into the temple' sensation; aversion to tobacco; light sleep; lack of sleep following worries or anxieties; sudden jumps while asleep.

Indications: **ANTIDOTE TO TOBACCO – INSOMNIA**

IPECA (Ipecac)

Symptoms: Mucous and glairy ('white of egg') vomiting preceded by waves of nausea and bringing no relief; intense salivation with clean tongue.

Indications: **VOMITING IN PREGNANCY.**

K

KALI BICHROMICUM (Potassium bichromate)

Symptoms: Racking and resounding cough which starts in the larynx; hoarse voice; yellowish and viscous (sticky) phlegm; retrosternal (behind the breast bone) pain ascending to the shoulders.

Indications: **COUGHS.**

KALI BROMATUM (Potassium bromide) *Symptoms*: Night terrors with cries and moans; sudden waking with fright.
Indications: **NIGHTMARES.**

L

LYCOPODIUM (Wolf's-foot, Wolf's-claw, Club-moss)
Symptoms: Extreme sensitivity; sudden outbursts of anger; difficulty in finding the right word; confusion in words and syllables; old-looking appearance of the child; ravenous hunger, but replete from the first mouthfuls; feeling of fullness in the stomach and abdomen.
Indications: **AGGRESSIVENESS – DYSLEXIA – LACK OF APPETITE.**

M

MELILOTUS (Melilot)
Symptoms: Nose-bleeding preceded by a redness of the face and a rush of blood to the head; throbbing of the carotids (neck arteries).
Indications: **NOSE-BLEEDING.**
MERCURIUS CYANATUS (Cyanide of mercury)
Symptoms: Thick, greyish coating on the mucous membrane of the mouth; tongue white with foetid breath.
Indications: **THRUSH.**
MERCURIUS SOLUBILIS (Soluble mercury)
Symptoms: Tongue swollen, yellowish, and retaining the imprint of the teeth; sore throat tending to suppurate; profuse salivation and foetid smell from the mouth; profuse night sweats; painful swelling of the parotid (beside the ear) glands.
Indications: **TONSILLITIS – MUMPS.**
MEZEREUM (Mezereon)
Symptoms: Ulcerations of the skin with purulent secretion, covered with yellowish scabs and surrounded by fiery and pruriginous vesicles (itchy blisters).
Indications: **IMPETIGO.**
MILLEFOLIUM (Achillea millefolium, Milfoil, Yarrow)
Symptoms: Haemorrhage of bright-red blood from the nose, either spontaneous or following a knock or blow on the face.
Indications: **NOSE-BLEEDING.**

MYRISTICA SEBIFERA (Otoba, Nutmeg)

Symptoms: Formation of boils or abscesses; speeds up the bursting of the pocket of pus.

Indications: **ABSCESS – BOIL.**

N

NATRUM MURIATICUM (Sodium chloride)

Symptoms: Emaciation and delayed development; tendency to get depressed and seek solitude; tendency to sulk; headaches characterized by violent throbs like hammer blows.

Indications: **GROWING PAINS.**

NITRIC ACID

Symptoms: Big warts with stalks on the back of the hands and bleeding when getting washed.

Indications: **WARTS.**

NUX VOMICA (Poison-nut)

Symptoms: Weight on the stomach with distension after meals; abdomen taut, swollen, and painful; vomiting of stomach contents often difficult to produce.

Indications: **INDIGESTION.**

P

PERTUSSINUM (Whooping-cough sputum)

Indications: **WHOOPING-COUGH.**

PETROLEUM

Symptoms: Oozing skin eruptions with pruriginous (itchy) and fiery vesicles (blisters) which leave behind clear running sores forming yellowish crusts.

Indications: **INFANTILE ECZEMA.**

PHOSPHORIC ACID

Symptoms: Impairment of memory in the pupil overworked at school; incapable of linking two ideas together.

Indications: **LOSS OF MEMORY.**

PLANTAGO (Plantain)

Symptoms: Nocturnal incontinence of urine.

Indications: **NOCTURNAL ENURESIS.**

PULSATILLA (Anemone pulsatilla, Pasque-flower)

Symptoms: Thick, yellowish, non-irritant secretions; right nostril blocked; reduced sense of smell.

Indications: **ADENOID GROWTHS**

Q

QUERCUS GLANDIUM SPIRITUS (Acorn)

Symptoms: Congestion of the head with hot flushes; tendency to dizziness.

Indications: **EXCESS OR ABUSE OF ALCOHOL.**

R

RHODODENDRON (Alpine rose)

Symptoms: Hypersensitivity to the raising of the electrical charge in the atmosphere; dread of thunder.

Indications: **FEAR OF THUNDERSTORMS.**

RHUS TOXICODENDRON (Poison sumac)

Symptoms: Skin red and puffy; presence of fiery swellings, soothed by heat; eruption of pruriginous (itchy) blisters.

Indications: **BURNS – CHICKEN-POX.**

S

SABINA (Savin, Juniper)

Symptoms: Tendency, at the least movement, to lose bright blood intermingled with clots from the womb; violent abdominal pains from the pubis (above external genitals) to the sacrum (composite bone at base of spine).

Indications: **RISK OF MISCARRIAGE.**

SAMBUCUS NIGRA (Common elder)

Symptoms: Sudden waking at night with a feeling of suffocation; cyanosis (blue coloration) of the face and extremities; impossibility of lying with the head low.

Indications: **INFANTILE ASTHMA.**

SENNA

Symptoms: The breath has an aromatic smell; attacks of nausea and vomiting with yellowish diarrhoea.

Indications: **KETONAEMIA.**

SILICEA (Silica)

Symptoms: Rickets; thinness; slow in walking; irritability; somnambulism; restless sleep; enlarged tonsils, especially on the left with a pricking sensation as if a needle had been stuck into this organ; pain on swallowing; enlargement of the lymphoid tissues in the form of a severe attack of asthma following repeated and poorly tolerated inoculations.

Indications: **TONSILLITIS – ADENOID GROWTHS – PYORRHOEA ALVEOLARIS (PARODONTAL DISEASE) – SLEEP-WALKING – DELAYED CLOSURE OF THE FONTANELLES – ANTIDOTE TO INOCULATIONS.**

STAPHYSAGRIA (Stavesacre)

Symptoms: Inflammation of the corner of the eye, which is pruriginous (itchy) and the site of small abscesses.

Indications: **STYES.**

STRAMONIUM (Thorn-apple)

Symptoms: Spasmodic constriction of the oesophagus (gullet) preventing swallowing.

Indications: **HICCUPS.**

SULPHUR IODATUM (Sulphur iodide)

Symptoms: Self-poisoning in women with tubercular heredity; chronic hypertrophy (overgrowth) of the tonsils; cervical adenopathies (neck swellings); skin irritations; tendency to herpes (skin eruption).

Indications: **HEREDITARY TAINTS – GANGLIA.**

T

TARAXACUM (Dandelion)

Symptoms: Coated tongue that looks like a map; sensation of abdominal fullness; regular constipation in the liverish child.

Indications: **CONSTIPATION.**

THUJA (White cedar)

Symptoms: Formation of burning and moist average-sized warts which bleed easily; brittle nails; adverse effects of vaccination.

Indications: **WARTS – ANTIDOTE TO VACCINATIONS.**

U

URTICA URENS (Stinging-nettle)

Symptoms: Superficial burns with skin irritations.

Indications: **BURNS.**

APPENDIX

Homoeopathic Hospitals
The following provide facilities within the National Health Service:

The Royal London Homoeopathic Hospital
Great Ormond Street, London WC1N 3HR
(Tel. 01-837 3091)

The Bristol Homoeopathic Hospital
Cotham Road, Cotham, Bristol BS6 6JU
(Tel. 0272 33068)

The Glasgow Homoeopathic Hospital
1000 Great Western Road, Glasgow G12 0NR
(Tel. 041-339 0382)

Outpatients Department
5 Lynedoch Crescent, Glasgow G3
(Tel. 041-332 4490)

The Tunbridge Wells Homoeopathic Hospital
Church Road, Tunbridge Wells, Kent
(Tel. 0892 42977)

The Liverpool Clinic
Department of Homoeopathy
Myrtle Street, Liverpool L7 7DE
(Tel. 051-709 8474)

Homoeopathic Clinics
Surgeries are held by homoeopathic doctors at the following clinics, but it is necessary to telephone for an appointment:

Berkshire -- 11 Hamilton Road, Reading
(Tel. Reading 883158 between 6.00 and 7.00 p.m.)

Berkshire -- The Priory, Binfield, Nr Bracknell
(Tel. 0344 3417)

Channel Islands -- Monthly visit. Contact Mrs Stievenard
(Tel. Jersey 42730)

Essex -- Thursday afternoons at The Surgery, Queen's Road,
Earl's Colne, Nr Colchester
(Tel. Earl's Colne 2022)

Hampshire -- Wednesday and Thursday (9.00 to 4.30 p.m.) at
Winchester Clinic, Bereweeke Road, Winchester
(Tel. 01-262 9745 or Winchester 64743)

Hampshire -- 20 Cliddesden Road, Basingstoke
(Tel. 0202 708180 or 0256 26590)

Isle of Wight -- Periodically at
29 Victoria Avenue, Shanklin
(Tel. Shanklin 2306)

Kent -- Periodically at
The Surgery, 12 Balmoral Road, Gillingham
(Tel. 0634 54933)

Leicester -- Leicester Homoeopathic Clinic,
193 Narborough Road, Leicester
(Tel. 548593)

London NW1 -- Weekdays (10.00 a.m. to 6.00 p.m.) at
6 Glentworth Street
(Tel. 01-486 8268)

London W1 -- 21/23 Seymour Street
(Tel. 01-723 8163 or 01-743 6310)

Manchester -- Daily at Brunswick Street, Ardwick
(Tel. 061-273 2446)

Middlesex -- 243 The Broadway, Southall
(Tel. 574 4281)

Somerset -- 49 Lyngford Road, Taunton
(Tel. Taunton 86251)

Suffolk -- c/o Mr David White, 56 Friars Street, Sudbury
(Tel. 0787 71404 or 73033)

Surrey -- 128 Great Tattenhams, Epsom Downs
(Tel. Burgh Heath 53660 day. Night and weekends 01-567 7326)

Sussex -- Most Tuesdays at 162 Goring Road, West Worthing
(Tel. Croydon 0534)

Sussex -- Twice monthly at
Stockbridge House, 26 Stockbridge Road, Chichester
(Tel. Chichester 782890)

Homoeopathic Chemists

A. Nelson & Co., 73 Duke Street, London W1M 6BY
(Tel. 01-629 3118)

E. Gould & Sons, 14 Crowndale Road, London NW1
(Tel. 01-388 4752)

Kilburn Chemists Ltd., 211 Belsize Road, London NW6
(Tel. 01-328 1030)

Stewarts Pharmacy, 59 Sheen Lane, London SW14
(Tel. 01-876 1861)

Galen Pharmacy, 1 South Terrace, South Street,
Dorchester, Dorset
(Tel. 0305 3996)

Weleda (UK) Ltd., Heanor Road, Ilkeston, Derbyshire DE7 8DR
(Tel. 0602 303151)

Platt's Chemists, 227 Seaview Road, Wallasey, Merseyside
(Tel. 051-639 1914)

Freemans, 7 Eaglesham Road, Clarkston, Glasgow

GENERAL CLINICAL INDEX

Other recommended books . . .

HOMOEOPATHIC PRESCRIBING

Remedies for Home and Surgery

Adolf Voegeli M.D. Written both for doctors wishing to learn something about this form of treatment, and for the layman who wants to use the remedies in the home, this book provides homoeopathic remedies based on symptoms and mental states, for many common ailments including 'flu, head colds, fevers, rheumatism, teething troubles, gastric upsets, etc. Homoeopathy is the perfect alternative to antibiotics since it does not produce any of the side effects associated with the latter. Not only are diseases quickly cured by homoeopathy; relapses seldom occur because the remedies strengthen the body's defensive powers.

THE ACUPUNCTURE TREATMENT OF PAIN

Leon Chaitow. *Large format Over 200 diagrams* For all who practise pain relief—doctors, surgeons, osteopaths, chiropractors, physiotherapists, trained nurses—this book shows how to apply the analgesic (pain relieving) and anaesthetic benefits of acupuncture with maximum efficacy. The location and anatomical position of each point is clearly described and given its Chinese name, traditional meridian name, and number. This information is adjacent to detailed, two-colour diagrams, thus enabling each point to be found with ease and accuracy. Author studied acupuncture under Dr. J. Lavier, and since 1966 he has researched into the usefulness of acupuncture for pain relief.

ARNICA

The Amazing Healer

A. C. Gordon Ross, M.F.Hom. Explains how the incredibly versatile Arnica, and twelve other 'vulneraries'—homoeopathic remedies known for their efficacy in healing wounds and other accident casualties—can benefit bruises, cuts, sprains, insect bites, and conditions such as sciatica, rheumatism, gout and back pain. Arnica is a quick-acting remedy for easing external wounds and mental upsets produced by bad news or sudden fright. Patients undergoing surgery are advised to take it before and after the operation. Includes a chapter on homoeopathic treatment for animals and provides a list of homoeopathic chemists, clinics and hospitals in England and Scotland.

PROVEN REMEDIES

The Treatment of Common Ailments by Homoeopathic, Herbal & Biochemic Methods

J. H. Oliver N.A.M.H. All these remedies are more genuinely scientific than drugs. The latter come and go, being first acclaimed and often ultimately discredited. But the herb and plant remedies endure: 'what cured a hundred years ago still cures today.' Here is a large number of alphabetically listed ailments, with the corresponding remedies and precise instructions as to dosage. In some cases osteopathy or chiropractic is also recommended and J. H. Oliver has added some valuable notes on deficiency foods, natural food, vitamins and germs.

HELPING YOURSELF WITH HOMOEOPATHIC REMEDIES

James H. Stephenson, M.D. A doctor reveals homoeopathic treatments used to bring *fast* relief to his own patients. There are sections on respiratory diseases, digestive tract upsets, bone and joint diseases, feminine ailments, skin problems, nervous troubles, sexual health problems, childhood ailments, allergies, and heart troubles. Now you can use specially energized dilutions of safe and natural substances to alleviate literally dozens of illnesses! Includes alphabetical list of homoeopathic medicines and the ailments that can be treated by each, plus alphabetical symptom guide.

EMERGENCY HOMOEOPATHIC FIRST-AID

A Quick Reference Handbook
Paul Chevanon M.D. & Rene Levannier M.D. The bedside book which no household should be without! Explains how to find immediate homoeopathic treatment for emergency illness while awaiting the doctor's arrival. Contains alphabetical listing of conditions and appropriate homoeopathic remedies. In addition there is a concise explanation of homoeopathy—its rules—homoeopathic dilutions and how they are made—the law of similarity. Homoeopathy treats the person rather than the disease, providing safe remedies which are invariably free from poisonous side effects!

PRESS POINT THERAPY

Gerard J. Bendix. *Illustrated.* Help yourself (and others) banish the pain of backache, headache, sinus, haemorrhoids, etc., by manipulating press points in the feet. These mark nerve-like connecting pathways leading to all parts of the body and are connector points to vital glands nerves and organs! Manipulation of these points can also delay the signs and effects of ageing—prevent oncoming or existing poor states of health—discover potential health complications almost before they occur—relieve nervous tension—and provide a quick energizer. You will be amazed how quickly you will locate the press points in your own—or somebody else's—feet. As you start feeling the beneficial effects, Press Point Therapy grows on you. The results speak for themselves!

CHINESE MICRO-MASSAGE

Acupuncture Without Needles

J. Lavier. *Illustrated.* Bridging the gap between classical massage and acupuncture micro-massage activates tiny points below the skin—either by hand or special instruments—and this action produces amazingly therapeutic results! It is an ideal therapy for squeamish patients or children who are afraid of having their flesh punctured, even minutely, by acupuncture needles. Although the *mechanical* action of micro-massage is feeble compared to massage proper, its uniquely *energizing* effect may be likened to the stimulation electrologists impart to muscles by the application of small electrodes. *Includes:* General technique; How to use the massage-points; Treatment of rheumatism.